Gastric Sleeve Cookbook+ Gastric Sleeve Diet

A step by step Food Guide for your Gastric Sleeve Surgery Recuperation. Planning What Eat Before and After Your Surgery with healthy foods. 2 books in 1

Alex Martinez

Gastric Sleeve Cookbook

A step by step Food Guide for your
Gastric Sleeve Surgery Recuperation.
Learn how to make easy Meal and
Recipes to Eat Well & Healthy. A Practical
Guide to Maximize Your Weight Loss
Results.

Alex Martinez

Contents

Introduction

A gastric sleeve is sometimes utilized as a treatment for obesity. Your physician performs with a laparoscopic sleeve gastrectomy, which can be an effective and minimally invasive bariatric surgery.

Laparoscopic sleeve gastrectomy -- only called a gastric sleeve surgery -- is a minimally invasive bariatric surgery employed in treating obesity and is currently being provided as a standalone process of morbidly obese patients. Patients have been carefully chosen to get a lap sleeve, and it's relatively secure with minimum risks even for high-risk sufferers. Be aware that vitamin and mineral nutritional supplements have to be used over longer intervals subsequent to the surgery.

Process.The gastric sleeve process eliminates the lateral two-thirds of their gut, which can be reduced using a stapling device. It's usually done laparoscopically to be able to be as minimally invasive as possible, and isn't reversible. The process essentially leaves a tummy tube in lieu of a stomach pouch.

The outcomes of weight loss surgeries change from 1 individual to another, and it's necessary to not forget that the outcomes may also be attributed to different factors like age, weight before surgery, exercise level, metabolism, and eating customs. Broadly, patients may lose 33 percent to 83 percent of excess body fat. Most of all, it is dependent upon your general commitment to a different lifestyle, which is ultimately what's going to help you shed weight, feel better, and improve your overall quality of life.

Chapter 1 what is gastric sleeve surgery? How it helps to reduce weight?

The Laparoscopic Sleeve Gastrectomy (LSG) is a Prohibitive Procedure that eliminates approximately 70 to 80 per cent of their gut. This leaves the gut in the form of a tube or "sleeve", about the size and form of a hot dog. This is an extremely successful weight reduction procedure which leads to hormonal changes that decrease appetite. The hormonal disturbance lasts for approximately a year, and then the little tubing of the gut limits food consumption.

The surgery doesn't involve rerouting of the intestines or implantation of artificial devices. The information available shows the Sleeve (LSG) to get overall weight reduction marginally lower compared to the Roux n Y Gastric bypass. Significant complications with this surgery are much like this

Roux n Y Gastric Bypass.

WeightWise is a program That's built to help individuals meet Their weight loss goals with achievement. This program is just for men and women that are thinking about changing their lifestyles and working through the whole program. The gastric sleeve procedure together with WeightWise takes patience, patience, and devotion.

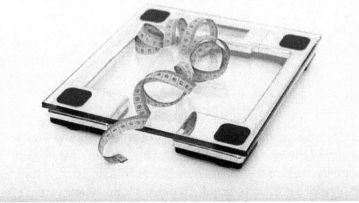

Prior to the procedure, patients are expected to attend least one service group meeting per month before surgery, but we invite each individual to attend as frequently as possible. These meetings provide you the chance to remain accountable to other people that are walking the exact same road as possible, and it plays a major part in your long-term weight loss success.

People who should think about the Gastric Sleeve process include the following:

• People who are worried about the possible long-term unwanted effects of an intestinal bypass.

• People who are worried about a foreign object within the

abdomen (ring).

• People who should always take anti inflammatory medications.

Pre-Operation Information

For most bariatric surgeries, the process begins weeks prior to the surgery. There's the first medical evaluation, emotional display, dialog with dietitians and exercise physiologists, and sleep test. All this is done in order to create certain to know everything that goes to a gastric sleeve surgery and other bariatric procedures.

Medical Analysis

That is if you meet the physicians to get an overview of your existing health and exploring which procedure is ideal for you. Not every customer is in precisely the exact same circumstance and no process is 1 size fits all. In this test, any healthcare problems -- past and present -- will be addressed.

We will also speak about your bodily history as a whole. Have you tried dieting or exercising previously? What worked and what did not? Were there major traumas or life events which obtained in the way of you living a healthy lifestyle? This will aid WeightWise craft the ideal weight loss plan for you.

Psychological Screening

In Weight Wise, We would like to make Sure That You Are physically as Well as emotionally prepared for gastric sleeve surgery. There's more to these processes than coming in, have the process, and then departing. We need to be certain to know what's going to happen for you along with your physique.

This is a large life time for our patients. The body will Experience a huge change, so your lifestyle will require a large shift, also. We would like to be certain that you're in the ideal place mentally for your surgery and allow you to work through any roadblocks you might have.

Dietitian Consult

Even though the gastric sleeve will limit your food Intake, it's likely to damage or even injure yourself if you deviate from the brand new lifestyle. Our dietitians will talk about beyond eating habits, nutritional expertise, and trigger factors that negatively affect your food intake. They'll also outline a strategy for the remainder of your life.

Sounds overwhelming, does not it? It does not need to be. After you know why you are doing so, it'll be a lot easier to find yourself eating less, getting more healthful, and feeling better than you have in quite a very long time. We are going to demonstrate how it is still possible to enjoy food whilst eating less of it.

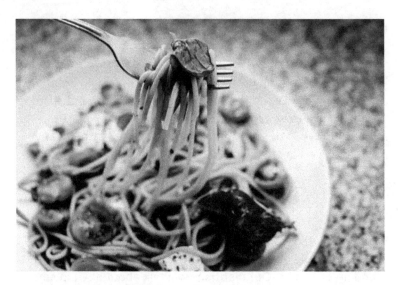

Incorporating Physical Activity

Even though the gastric sleeve process and enhancing your eating Customs are surely great ways to drop weight, instituting a workout regimen can allow you to keep off the weight. Are you going to have to run three miles daily and hit the weights? Certainly not!

Our exercise physiologists will outline a schedule especially for you personally and go over both short- and - long term objectives. Although, if among these goals occurs to comprise running a marathon or turning into a power lifter, we could help you achieve those peaks. However, improving your cardiovascular system, flexibility, and total strength are the chief concerns.

Sleep Assessment

Ultimately, We'll Speak to you about sleep apnea and the way it can impact the achievement of the gastric sleeve surgery both during and following the procedure. We need this lifestyle shift to function as far as you can do, therefore we'll research if you suffer from sleep apnea or not.

All this is to Make Certain You have all of the information you Need to create this very important choice. Weight Wise needs all our patients to live long, productive lives well following the gastric sleeve surgery. That is why those consultations are so significant -- the more people understand about our patients; the greater it's before, during, and following the process.

Post Operation Information

When the surgery is complete and after a night of Monitoring, you're free to come back to your regular activities. Grocery shopping, playing with your children, or simply walking around the area -- maybe for the first time in a very long time -- is not off-limits. You may go back to work based on the type of job you've got.

Working behind a desk is nice, but you Might Want to take a Couple more days prior to returning to this building job. We urge people who have tasks that need physical exertion speak with their supervisors about easing back in the position. And as you might be prepared to come back to daily tasks, it is important to keep in mind that you cannot return to a previous lifestyle.

This is where the actual work starts. The discussions, the Diets, and everything that occurred in the months or weeks leading up to the gastric sleeve process were to prepare one for right now. The surgery is only 1 step on the long trip to health. Remember: each circumstance differs! The following is only 1 instance of a post-op diet.

Learning How to Eat Properly

In fourteen days after the surgery, your food consumption will be restricted to largely fluids. It is important to remain hydrated at this stage and give your body the electrolytes it requires. You'll also receive protein nutritional supplements to round out your dietplan. It is ideal to steer clear of liquids with sugar or caffeine in this time.

Do not gulp the liquid! It could be too much strain on the Sleeve along with your physique. Take modest sips till you learn just how much you are able to take in 1 swig. This diet is designed to get your entire body in tune with all the new food ingestion. Hormones in your body will start adapting to the diet and you will start to feel fuller faster.

Soft proteins have been introduced between four and two months as Your own body continues to adapt to a new lifestyle. This usually means no protein supplements or pureed foods, possibly. It is still extremely important to hydrate in this time. Deviating in the diet may lead to pain, distress, and even harm. In rare situations, it might even alter the surgery itself, undoing all of the work that you put in prior.

After four weeks, then you will Have the Ability to expand your diet more. Lean proteins, non-starchy veggies, along with other food according to your dietitian. Carbs are a huge no-no for many individuals, as are sweet and fattening foods. We know it sounds hard, but you came to us to make a lifestyle change -- that is exactly what it requires.

However, you will not be lonely. Our individual urges are that you Response questions, assist you through rough patches, and provide you the encouragement you will need to find that all of the way through. Think of these as your personal cheerleaders!

Break a sweat

The Majority of our gastric Sleeve processes are done laparoscopically, and it is a set of small incisions. These tiny incisions heal much quicker compared to one long incision which has been used previously, meaning downtime was reduced greatly. So you are in a position to return to normal activities almost immediately.

Included in this pre-op program, exercise physiologists and Patients discuss what sort of exercise program ought to be utilized after the surgery. Determined by flexibility, cardiovascular, and strength, Weight Wise considers in the "Work Smart, Not Harder" axiom. Many individuals have back, hip, or knee difficulties as a result of excessive weight. All this is taken into consideration when organizing a program.

As endurance and strength start to grow, the workouts will be adjusted to make the most of this progress. But, there's actually no "endpoint" when it comes to physical action. Exercise is just as essential as eating healthy, both to your body and the brain.

Undergoing the gastric sleeve process is a huge deal for a lot of folks, and our highly trained staff of specialists in Weight Wise knows that you may feel overwhelmed. We're here in order to answer your questions and set your mind at ease! There is nothing better than getting your self-confidence back! That assurance is simply one of the wonderful components of getting this surgery and can be a byproduct of having a human body which you adore and have worked hard for you.

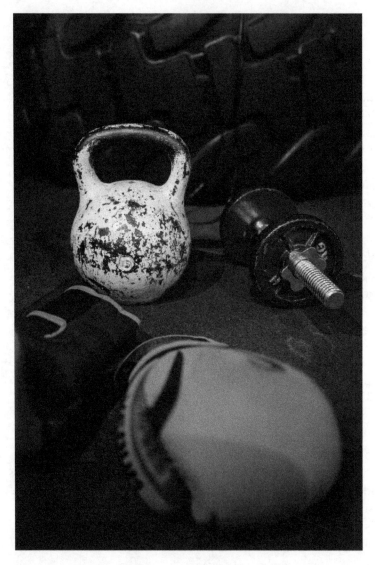

Things to Know About Gastric Sleeve Weight Loss Surgery

1 approach to tackle obesity would be with regular surgery. This
Kind of surgery involves removing or diminishing the size of
your tummy. Bariatric surgery typically contributes to rapid

weight reduction.

Gastric sleeve surgery is one of several Kinds of bariatric Surgery choices. Medical professionals typically call it vertical sleeve gastrectomy.

In this Guide, you'll have a closer look at what is involved in gastric sleeve surgery, such as its efficacy and potential complications.

What exactly does gastric sleeve surgery demand?

Gastric sleeve surgery is almost always performed as a invasive procedure using a laparoscope. This usually means a very long, thin tube is inserted into your abdomen through several tiny incisions. This tube has a light and a small camera attached to it and many tools.

Gastric sleeve surgery is performed with general anesthesia, which is medication that puts you right into a really deep sleep and takes a ventilator to breathe for you during the surgery.

The surgery involves dividing your gut into 2 unequal Components. Approximately 80 percent of those outer curved portion of your gut is cut off and removed.

The advantages of the remaining 20 percent are then stapled or sutured together. This produces a banana-shaped stomach that is just about 25% of its initial size.

You are going to be at the living room about one hour. After the Surgery is finished, you're going to be moved into the recovery area for health care. You are going to be at the recovery area for one more hour or so as you awaken from the anesthesia.

The tiny incisions in your abdomen typically cure fast. The

minimally invasive nature of this surgery makes it possible to recuperate faster than a process where your stomach is started using a bigger incision.

Unless there are complications, you should have the Ability to go Home within two or three days following the surgery

Is it successful?

Gastric sleeve surgery helps you Eliminate weight in two manners:

• Your Stomach is considerably smaller in order to feel full and stop eating earlier. As a result, that you take in fewer calories.

• The component Of the stomach that generates ghrelin -- a hormone that is connected with appetite -- has been eliminated, which means you are much less hungry.

According to the American Society of Metabolic and Allergic Surgery, you can expect to lose at least 50 per cent of your extra weight over the 18 to 24 weeks after gastric sleeve surgery. Some folks lose 60 to 70 percent Trusted Source.

It is Important to Keep in Mind that this Is Only Going to happen if you Are dedicated to adhering to the diet and exercise plan recommended by the physician. By embracing these lifestyle modifications, you are more inclined to keep the weight off long term.

Who's a fantastic candidate for this surgery?

Bariatric surgery of any type, such as gastric sleeve Surgery, is just considered a choice when powerful attempts to boost your diet and exercise habits, and also the usage of weight-loss drugs, have not worked.

Even after that, you have to meet specific standards to be eligible for A regular procedure. These standards are based on the own body mass index (BMI) and if you have some obesity-related wellness conditions.

Qualifying conditions:

• Intense (morbid) obesity (BMI rating of 40 or greater)

• Obesity (BMI rating of 35 to 39) with one important obesity-related condition

Sometimes, gastric sleeve surgery is completed if you are Obese but do not fulfill the standards for obesity, however, you get a substantial health condition associated with your weight.

What are the complications and risks?

Gastric sleeve surgery is known as a relatively safe procedure. But like all significant surgeries, there may be dangers and complications.

Some complications may happen after any surgery. All these include:

• Hemorrhage. Bleeding in the wound or within your body may result in shock when it is severe.

• Deep vein thrombosis (DVT). Surgery as well as the healing procedure can boost your chance of a blood clot forming on your vein, usually in a leg vein.

• Pulmonary embolism. A pulmonary embolism can occur when a part of a blood clot breaks off and travels to your lungs.

• Irregular heartbeat. Surgery may boost the danger of an irregular pulse, particularly atrial fibrillation.

• Pneumonia. Pain can permit you to take shallow breaths that may result in a lung disease, such as pneumonia.

Gastric sleeve surgery may have added complications. A few possible side effects that are specific to this surgery include:

• Gastric leaks. Stomach fluids can flow in the suture line on your gut where it had been stitched back together.

• Stenosis. Section of your gastric sleeve may shut, resulting in an obstruction in your stomach.

• Vitamin deficiencies. The part of your gut that is eliminated is partially responsible for the absorption of vitamins that your body needs. If you don't take vitamin supplements, then this may result in deficiencies.

• Heartburn (GERD). Reshaping your gut can cause or aggravate heartburn. This may normally be treated with over-the-counter drugs.

It is Important to Keep in Mind that changing your diet and Exercise habits are crucial to losing the weight and keeping it off following gastric sleeve surgery. It is potential to gain the weight back if you

• eat also much

• consume an unhealthy diet

• exercise too little

Other concerns

Another Frequent concern, especially Once You Get Rid of Lots of Weight fast, is that the massive number of surplus skin you might be left with as the pounds drop away. This is a frequent complication of gastric sleeve surgery.

This excess skin could be removed if it disturbs you. But remember it may take around 18 months for the body to stabilize following gastric sleeve surgery. That is why it's generally better to wait until considering a skin removal process. Until then, you might want to try out some strategies for tightening loose skin.

Another thing to think about before choosing to have gastric Sleeve surgery is that, unlike any other regular surgeries, gastric sleeve surgery is permanent. If you aren't satisfied with the outcome, your tummy cannot be transformed back to how it was.

How can your diet alter following gastric sleeve surgery?

Before gastric sleeve surgery is completed, you typically must consent to particular lifestyle modifications recommended by your physician. These changes are supposed to assist you reach and maintain weight loss.

One of these changes involves eating a healthy diet for the remainder of your life.

Your physician will recommend the very best gastric sleeve diet to get you after your surgery. The dietary modifications your surgeon proposes may be like the overall dietary guidelines under.

Dietary changes

• Two weeks Prior surgery. Boost protein, lower carbs, and remove sugar from the dietplan.

• Two days before and the first week following surgery. Ingest only clear fluids which are caffeine- and - carbonation-free.

• For the Next three months. It's possible to add pureed food into your diet plan.

You will usually have the Ability to eat regular, Healthful food about 1 month following your surgery. You might discover that you just eat less than prior to the process since you will get full fast and will not feel overly hungry.

Your restricted diet and smaller foods may cause some Nutritional deficiencies. It is important to compensate for this by choosing multivitamins, calcium supplements, a monthly B-12 shot, and many others as recommended by your physician.

Is it covered by insurance?

In the USA, most health insurers realize that obesity is a risk factor for other health conditions that may result in serious medical issues. Because of this, many insurance businesses cover gastric sleeve surgery when you've got a qualifying state.

In accordance with the Centers of Medicare & Medicare Services (CMS), Medicare will cover gastric sleeve surgery if you meet the following requirements:

• Your BMI Is 35 or greater

• You've one or more obesity-related health ailments

• You had been not able to eliminate the weight by simply modifying your diet and exercise habits or simply by taking drugs

Medicare does not cover gastric sleeve surgery in case you are Obese but do not possess an obesity-related health state.

Without health insurance policy, the price of gastric Sleeve surgery may vary widely from 1 area into another, and also from 1 centre to another in the exact same geographical location. Normally, the price could range from $15,000 to over $25,000.

Given this wide variation, it is Ideal to study and Speak to Several operative and surgeons facilities to find one you are comfortable with -- and also one which satisfies your budget.

The Main Point

Gastric sleeve surgery is one of several Kinds of bariatric Surgery choices. It works by making your stomach smaller so that you eat less. Since the dimensions of the gut are reduced, you will also realize that you are less hungry.

To be eligible for gastric sleeve surgery, you need to meet specific criteria. You have to show that you have attempted other weight-loss strategies -- such as diet, exercise, and weight loss drugs -- with no success. Other qualifying standards comprise your BMI and if you have some obesity-related wellness conditions.

Should you follow a healthy diet and exercise regimen frequently after gastric sleeve surgery, you could have the ability to shed more than 50 per cent of your extra weight over 24 months.

However, as with the Majority of surgical procedures, there's the danger of side effects and complications. If you are considering gastric sleeve surgery, speak to your physician about whether you are eligible for this process and if it is a secure solution for you.

Chapter 2 Recipes for gastric sleeve!

Cajun Chicken Stuffed With Pepper Jack Cheese and Spinach Recipe

Weight Management & Bariatrics

SERVINGS: 4

INGREDIENTS

• 1 pound (16 oz) boneless, skinless chicken breasts

• 3 ounce reduced fat pepper jack cheese (Shredded)

• 1 cup frozen spinach thawed and drained (or fresh cooked)

• 2 tsp Olive oil

• 2 tablespoon Cajun seasoning (see recipe below if You Would like to Create homemade)

• 1 tablespoon bread crumbs

• Toothpicks

INSTRUCTIONS

1. Preheat Oven to 350º F levels.

2. Flatten the chicken into 1/4-inch thickness.

3. In a Medium bowl, combine the pepper jack cheese, spinach, salt and pepper.

4. Blend That the Cajun seasoning and breadcrumbs together in a little bowl.

5. Spoon Roughly 1/4 c of the spinach mixture onto each chicken breast. Roll each chicken breast fasten the seams with several toothpicks.

6. Brush every chicken breast with the olive oil. Distribute the Cajun seasoning mix evenly over all.

7. Sprinkle any residual spinach and cheese on top of chicken (optional).

8. set the Chicken seam-side up on a tin foil-lined baking sheet (for effortless cleanup).

9. Bake for 35 to 40 minutes or till chicken is cooked through.

10. Eliminate the toothpicks before serving. Hurry to ensure that you have eliminated every last toothpick.

11. Drink Entire or slice into medallions.

Cajun Seasoning (makes about 2 tbsp)

- 3/4 tablespoon paprika

- 3/4 tsp onion powder

- 3/4 tsp garlic powder

- 1/4 tsp Black pepper

- 1/2 tsp cayenne pepper

- 1/4 tsp White pepper

- 1/4 tsp cumin

- 1/4 tsp thyme

- 1/4 tsp oregano

NUTRITION FACTS

1 serving (4 servings per recipe)

Calories: 241

Total Fat: 9.7gram

Total Carbohydrates: 2g

Dietary Fiber: 1g

Sugars: 0g

Complete Protein: 32g

Chicken Rollantini using Spinach ala Parmigiana Recipe

Weight Management & Bariatrics

SERVINGS: 8

INGREDIENTS

8 chicken breast cutlets (pounded thin)--3 ounces each

1/2 cup whole wheat Italian seasoned breadcrumbs

1/4 cup grated parmesan cheese, divided

6 tbsp egg whites/egg beaters, split

5 ounces frozen spinach, thawed and squeezed dry of any liquid

6 tablespoon part skims ricotta cheese

6 ounces part skim mozzarella--shredded, divided

Non-stick cooking spray

1 cup marinara sauce

INSTRUCTIONS

1. Preheat Oven to 450º levels

2. Spray 9x13 glass baking dish with nonstop cooking spray.

3. Season Chicken cutlets with pepper & salt

4. In a Small bowl, combine breadcrumbs with two tbsp grated parmesan cheese.

5. Place 1/4 Cup egg whites in another bowl.

6. Blend 1.5 ounce mozzarella cheese with remaining grated parmesan cheese, spinach, remaining 2 tablespoons egg whites, and ricotta cheese.

7. Lay Experienced, pounded chicken cutlets on working surface

and disperse two tbsp of spinach-cheese combinations on each.

8. Loosely Roll each cutlet, maintaining the seam side down and fasten with a toothpick or 2.

9. Dip the Chicken rolls egg whites, then in breadcrumb mixture and put seam-side down in greased baking dish.

10. Duplicate with chicken.

11. Gently spray chicken rollantinis with non stick spray.

12. Bake 25 Minutes, or till instant-read thermometer reads 165°F.

13. Eliminate, Shirt with marinara sauce and staying mozzarella cheese.

14. Bake for 3 more moments, until cheese is melted and bubbling.

15. Serve with Extra sauce on the side and grated parmesan cheese.

NUTRITION FACTS

1 serving (~1 full breast)

Total calories: 268

Total fat: 9 g

Total carbohydrates: 8 grams

Dietary Fiber: 1.5 gram

Sugars: 3 g

Protein: 36 g

Cottage Cheese Fluff Recipe

Weight Management & Bariatrics

SERVINGS: 8

INGREDIENTS

Two 24-ounce containers skillet cottage cheese

1 8-ounce sugar-free whipped topping

Two 0.3-ounces packs sugar-free gelatin, taste of choice

DIRECTIONS

1. Mix all Ingredients in a big bowl.

2. Optional -- add your favorite fruit.

NUTRITIONAL ANALYSIS PER SERVING (1 serving is about 1 cup):

Total calories: 220

Total fat: 3 g

Total carbohydrates: 24 gram

Dietary Fiber: 0 grams

Sugars: 4 g

Protein: 22 g

Zucchini Boat Recipe

Weight Management & Bariatrics

SERVINGS: 8

INGREDIENTS

4 medium zucchini

1 lb ground turkey breast

1/2 cup sliced onion

1 egg, beaten

1/2 pounds chopped mushrooms

1 large tomato diced

3/4 cup skillet

1/4 cup experienced whole wheat bread crumbs

1/4 tsp salt

1/4 tsp pepper

1 cup (4 oz) shredded low fat mozzarella cheese

DIRECTIONS

1. Cut Zucchini in half lengthwise; cut a thin slice in the base of each using a sharp knife to permit zucchini to sit level.

2. Scoop out pulp, leaving 1/4-in. shells. Set pulp apart.

3. Place Cubes within an ungreased 3-qt. microwave-safe dish. Cover and microwave on high for 3 minutes or till crisp-tender; drain and put aside.

4. In a Large skillet, cook ground turkey and onion over moderate heat until meat is no longer pink; drain. Remove from heat.

5. In a Large bowl blend together zucchini pulp, crushed egg, skillet, bread crumbs, mushrooms, tomato, pepper, salt, 1/2 cup cheese and cooked ground turkey.

6. Spoon roughly 1/4 cup mixture into each shell.

7. Sprinkle with cheese.

8. Bake Found for 20 minutes in 350º F or till brown.

NUTRITIONAL ANALYSIS PER SERVING (1 zucchini ship or 1/8 Recipe):

Total Calories: 195

Total Fat: 7.5gram

Saturated Fat: 3g

Sodium: 294 mg

Total Carbohydrates: 16g

Dietary Fiber: 4g

Sugars: 5g

Protein: 17.5g

Egg Muffin Recipe

Weight Management & Bariatrics

SERVINGS: 12

INGREDIENTS

6 large eggs

12 slices pre-cooked turkey bacon (chopped into thirds)

3/4 cup shredded low fat Swiss or Monterey jack cheese

1/2 cup 1 percent milk

1/4 tsp salt

1/4 tsp pepper

1/4 tsp Italian seasoning

DIRECTIONS

1. Spray muffin tin with nonstick cooking spray.

2. Preheat Oven to 350º F.

3. Place 3 Bacon pieces at the bottom of each muffin cup.

4. In a Separate bowlmix together all ingredients until well mixed, except for 1/4 cup of the shredded cheese.

5. Fill each Muffin cup with 1/4 cup of the egg mix.

6. Sprinkle Additional 1/4 cup of cheese in addition to muffins.

7. Bake for 20-25 minutes or till eggs are set.

NUTRITIONAL ANALYSIS PER SERVING (1 muffin):

Total Calories: 98

Total Fat: 7g

Saturated fat: 2g

Total Carbohydrates: 1g

Complete Fiber: 0g

Complete Sugar: 1g

Protein: 8g

Cottage Cheese Cake Recipe

Weight Management & Bariatrics

SERVINGS: 8

INGREDIENTS

2 cups low-fat or fat-free cottage cheese

2 whole eggs

10-ounce package of frozen spinach (thawed and drained)

1/2 cup Parmesan cheese

DIRECTIONS

1. Preheat Oven to 350° F.

2. In big Bowl, combine all ingredients together well.

3. Place Calmly into 8x8 pan.

4. Bake for 20-30 minutes or until cheese bubbles outside.

5. Let sit Minutes prior to serving.

6. Season to Flavor with pepper, salt, and garlic as wanted.

NUTRITIONAL ANALYSIS PER SERVING (roughly 1/2 cup):

Total calories: 78

Total fat: 3 g

Total carbohydrates: 3 gram

Dietary Fiber: 1 gram

Sugars: 2 g

Protein: 11 g

Cottage Cheese Cake Recipe

Weight Management & Bariatrics

SERVINGS: 8

INGREDIENTS

2 cups low-fat or fat-free cottage cheese

2 whole eggs

10-ounce package of frozen spinach (thawed and drained)

1/2 cup Parmesan cheese

DIRECTIONS

1. Preheat Oven to 350° F.

2. In big Bowl, combine all ingredients together well.

3. Place Calmly into 8x8 pans.

4. Bake for 20-30 minutes or until cheese bubbles outside.

5. Let sit Minutes prior to serving.

6. Season to Flavor with pepper, salt, and garlic as wanted.

NUTRITIONAL ANALYSIS PER SERVING (roughly 1/2 cup):

Total calories: 78

Total fat: 3 g

Total carbohydrates: 3 gram

Dietary Fiber: 1 gram

Sugars: 2 g

Protein: 11 g

Tofu and Broccoli Quiche Recipe

Weight Management & Bariatrics

SERVINGS: 6

INGREDIENTS

1/2 cup uncooked bulgur wheat

Pinch of salt

1 tbsp sesame oil

1 yellow onion, chopped

1/2 pound broccoli, sliced

1/4 pound mushrooms, sliced

11/2 pounds kale

2 tbsp sesame tahini

1 tablespoon umeboshi paste (pickled plum paste) or white miso

1 tbsp tamari

DIRECTIONS

1. Preheat oven to 350? F.

2. Bring 1 Cup water to a boil in a small pot, add bulgur and salt and then come back to a boil.

3. Lower heat, cover and cook for 15 minutes.

4. Press hot Bulgur to a greased 9-inch dish pan and boiled for 12 minutes, or till slightly dry and crust-like. Put aside.

5. Heat oil at a large skillet over medium heat.

6. Insert Onions, celery, broccoli and mushrooms to skillet and cook briefly.

7. Cover Skillet and turn heat off; set aside while you prepare kale mixture.

8. Combination tofu, tahini, umeboshi paste and tamari in a food processor until smooth.

9. Transfer Mix into a bowl and then add fruits. Toss gently to blend.

10. Pour Vegetable mix into bulgur crust, and then bake for half an hour.

11. Eliminate from oven and let sit 10 minutes.

12. Cut into 6 Slices pieces and serve hot or cold.

NUTRITIONAL ANALYSIS PER SERVING (⅙ recipe):

Total Calories: 190

Total Fat: 8g

Saturated fat: 1 gram

Total cholesterol: 0 milligrams

Sodium: 350 mg

Total carbohydrates: 18g

Dietary fiber: 4g

Sugar: 3g

Protein: 13g

Faux Fried Chicken Recipe

Weight Management & Bariatrics

SERVINGS: 3

INGREDIENTS

1/3 cup reduced-fat buttermilk

⅛ Tsp. paprika

12 oz. raw boneless skinless lean chicken breast tenders (about 10 bits)

1/3 cup bran cereal (Original Fiber One® or similar kind)

1/3 cup panko breadcrumbs

1 Tbsp. Dry onion soup mix

Optional: salt, to taste

DIRECTIONS

1. In a Large sealable container or plastic bag, combine buttermilk with paprika and blend well.

2. Insert Chicken and coat completely. Seal and refrigerate for 1 hour.

3. Preheat Oven to 375 degrees.

4. Prepare a Big baking sheet by spraying it with non stick spray. Put aside.

5. Employing a Blender or food processor, grind cereal into some breadcrumb-like consistency. Pour crumbs into a large bowl.

6. Insert panko breadcrumbs and onion soup mix. If you prefer, add a dash or two of salt. Mix thoroughly.

7. One in a Time, eliminate each piece of chicken out of container/bag, give it a shake (to eliminate surplus buttermilk), coat it evenly with the crumb mixture, and put it flat on the baking sheet.

8. Bake in The oven for 10 minutes. Switch carefully (tongs work well!)) , then bake for another 10 minutes, or until outsides are crispy and chicken is cooked through.

NUTRITIONAL ANALYSIS PER SERVING (1/3 recipe or roughly 3 Bits):

Total calories: 210

Total Fat: 3.5g

Total Carbohydrates: 17g

Complete Fiber: 3.5gram

Complete Sugar: 2g

Protein: 29g

Cheesy Vegetarian Chili Recipe

Weight Management & Bariatrics

SERVINGS: 8 (roughly 11/2 cups per day)

INGREDIENTS

2 garlic cloves

2 tsp olive oil

1 large green bell pepper (diced)

1 cup onion chopped

1/2 pound of chopped mushrooms

14.5-ounce can of diced tomatoes or 2 cups fresh berries

8 oz tomato sauce

2 tbsp chili powder

1 medium zucchini (thinly sliced)

Two 15-ounce cans red kidney beans (rinsed)

10-ounce package of coriander

1 cup low fat shredded cheddar cheese

DIRECTIONS

1. Heating Olive oil and garlic in large pan.

2. Insert Onions, celery, green pepper, and mushrooms. Cook till tender.

3. Insert in Tomato sauce, diced tomatoes, chili powder, and bring to boil.

4. Switch down To low, include zucchini and kidney beans. Simmer for 10-15 minutes.

5. Insert frozen corn and 1/2 cup cheddar cheese. Stir.

6. Simmer on Low for extra 10-15 minutes.

7. Drink topped with cheddar cheese.

NUTRITIONAL ANALYSIS PER SERVING (roughly 11/2 cups)

Calories: 195

Total Fat: 3 g

Protein: 13 g

Total Carbohydrates: 34 g

Dietary Fiber: 9 g

Sugars: 6 g

Creamy Slow Cooker Chicken Recipe

Weight Management & Bariatrics

SERVINGS: 6

INGREDIENTS

6 skinless, boneless chicken breasts (two 1/2 pounds)

103/4 ounce reduced fat cream of mushroom soup

1 cup pureed cottage cheese or plain Greek yogurt

1/2 cup chicken stock

0.7 ounce Oven Italian dressing mix

8 oz pkg mushrooms

Cooking spray

DIRECTIONS

1. Spray a Big skillet with cooking spray. Cook chicken in batches within medium-high heat 2-3 minutes on each side or until just browned. Transfer chicken to a 5-qt. slow cooker.

2. Add soup, Cottage cheese or yogurt, chicken stock, and Italian dressing mix to skillet. Cook over moderate heat, stirring constantly, 2-3 minutes or till cheese is melted and mixture is smooth.

3. Arrange Mushrooms in slow cooker. Spoon soup mixture over mushrooms. Cover and cook on LOW 4 hours. Stir well before serving.

4. To create forward: Prepare recipe as directed. Transfer into a 13- x 9-inch baking dish, and let cool completely. Freeze up to a month. Thaw in refrigerator 8 to 24 hours. To reheat, cover tightly with aluminum foil, and bake at 325? For 45 minutes. Uncover and bake 15 minutes or until thoroughly warmed.

NUTRITIONAL ANALYSIS PER SERVING (1 six-ounce percentage):

Calories: 128

Protein: 18.5 g

Fat: 1.68 g

Sugar: 2.28 g

Cheesy Crustless Quiche Recipe

Weight Management & Bariatrics

SERVINGS: 8

INGREDIENTS

4 oz cubed infant low fat Swiss

6 oz broiled chicken breast, cut into 1" cubes

10 oz shredded low fat mozzarella cheese

3 large eggs

1 cup skim milk

Oregano to year (if wanted)

Nonstick cooking spray

9" pie pan

DIRECTIONS

1. Preheat Oven to 400 degrees.

2. Spray pie Pan with non stick cooking spray.

3. Fill the Pie pan together with the cubed infant Swiss and cubed chicken breastfeeding.

4. Spread the two cups of shredded mozzarella cheese on the top of the whole mixture.

5. Sprinkle the oregano on the top to taste.

6. In a Separate bowl, whip together the eggs and skim milk. Pour over the cheese and chicken.

7. Bake in 400 degrees for 40 minutes. (The top will probably be quite lightly browned when completed.)

8. Let cool and serve immediately or cover with tinfoil and put in fridge.

Feel free to add fruits to tastes -- tomatoes, onions, green pepper.

NUTRITIONAL ANALYSIS PER SERVING (⅛ quiche)

Calories: 176

Fat: 9 g

Carbohydrates: 3.6 gram

Sugar: 2 g

Protein: 19.5 g

Cheesy Stuffed Acorn Squash Recipe

Weight Management & Bariatrics

SERVINGS: 4

INGREDIENTS

2 acorn squash, halved and seeded

1 pounds (16 ounce) extra lean ground turkey breast

1 cup diced celery

1 cup finely chopped onion

1 cup fresh mushrooms, sliced

1 tsp basil

1 tsp oregano

1 tsp garlic powder

1/8 tsp salt

1 pinch ground black pepper

8 ounces can tomato sauce

1 cup low fat shredded Cheddar cheese

DIRECTIONS

1. Preheat Oven to 350 degrees F (175 degrees C).

2. Place Squash cut side down into a glass dish.

3. Cook in Microwave for 20 minutes on HIGH, until nearly tender.

4. In a Non-stick saucepan over moderate heat, brown ground turkey.

5. Insert celery and onion; sauté until transparent.

6. Stir in Mushrooms; cook two to three minutes longer.

7. Insert in Tomato sauce and dry seasonings

8. Split Mix into quarters, then spoon to the skillet and pay.

9. Cook 15 minutes in the preheated 350 degrees F (175 degrees C) oven.

10. Uncover, Scatter cheese and place back into the oven till the cheese bubbles.

NUTRITION ANALYSIS PER SERVING

Calories: 299

Total Fat: 4g

Total Carbohydrates: 38g

Dietary Fiber: 6g

Sugars: 9g

Complete Protein: 30g

Spicy Avocado Spread Recipe

Weight Management & Bariatrics

SERVINGS: 6

INGREDIENTS

1 ripe, darkened avocado

2/3 cup white or cannellini beans, rinsed and drained

2 ample sprigs of cilantro

1 1/2 Tablespoons fresh lime juice (1-2 limes)

1/2 green jalapeño, seeds removed and chopped

1/2 tsp green Tabasco sauce

1/4 tsp salt

DIRECTIONS

1. In a Blender or food processor combine all ingredients until creamy and smooth

2. Dip Vegetables to disperse or use as a topping on poultry

NUTRITIONAL ANALYSIS PER SERVING (3-4 tsp)

Calories: 85

Fat: 5 g

Protein: 2 g

Carbohydrate: 8 g

Fiber: 4 g

Sodium: 105 mg

Sugar: nominal

Fruity Breakfast Wrap Recipe

Weight Management & Bariatrics

SERVINGS: 1)

INGREDIENTS

1 whole wheat tortilla (little; 113kcal)

3 Tablespoons of Normal ricotta cheese

1 Tablespoon of low-sugar, strawberry jelly

1/3 cup fresh, chopped tomatoes

DIRECTIONS

1. Spread ricotta cheese and jelly on tortilla

2. Sprinkle Chopped tomatoes on top of ricotta cheese and jelly

3. Roll up Tortilla and revel in!

NUTRITIONAL ANALYSIS PER SERVING (1 tortilla wrap)

Calories: 233

Fat: 9 g

Protein: 8 g

Carbohydrate: 30 g

Cholesterol: 24 mg

Sodium: 229 mg

Sugar: 8 g

Creamy Cauliflower Puree Recipe

Weight Management & Bariatrics

SERVINGS: 4

INGREDIENTS

1 large (6 to 7 inches in diameter) head of cauliflower

3 cloves of garlic (cooked/steamed with cauliflower)

1/3 cup low-fat buttermilk

4 tsp extra-virgin olive oil

1 tsp butter, salted

1/2 tsp of garlic salt

1/2 tsp of black pepper

DIRECTIONS

1. Break Steak into 2" x 2" pieces (or smaller) and place in large microwave safe bowl using 1/4 cup water plus 3 whole garlic cloves and pay.

2. Microwave For 5 minutes or until cauliflower is very tender.

3. Use Garlic press to crush garlic cloves and add them into food processor. Add cooked cauliflower into your food processor.

4. Insert Buttermilk, 2 tsp olive oil, butter, garlic salt, and pepper.

5. Procedure Ingredients until creamy and smooth.

6. Drizzle the remaining two tsp of olive oil on top and serve.

NUTRITIONAL ANALYSIS PER SERVING (3/4 cup serving)

Calories: 113

Fat: 6 g

Protein: 5 g

Carbohydrate: 13 g

Cholesterol: 3 mg

Sodium: 383 mg

Sugar: 6 g

Provencal Chicken Slow-Cooker Recipe

Weight Management & Bariatrics

SERVINGS: 4

INGREDIENTS

2 boneless, skinless chicken breast halves, cut in half Lengthwise (about 1 1/2 lbs)

2 tsp dried basil

1/4 tsp salt

1/4 tsp black pepper

1 cup diced yellow bell pepper

1 (16-ounce) can navy beans, rinsed and drained

1 (14 1/2 oz) can diced tomatoes, undrained

Dried or fresh basil leaves (optional)

DIRECTIONS

1. Place chicken in an electric slow cooker or crockpot.

2. In a Large bowl, mix salt, black pepper, bell pepper, beans, tomatoes and dried ginger (if using fresh ginger, add in the end); stir well.

3. Spoon Mix over chicken.

4. Cook Low setting for 4-6 hours or until chicken reaches 165°F.

5. Drink each chicken breast with tomato and bean mixture spooned over the top.

6. Garnish with dried or fresh basil leaves, if desired.

NUTRITIONAL ANALYSIS PER SERVING (1/2 chicken breast and 3/4 cup Bean mix)

Calories: 315

Fat: 2 g

Protein: 38 g

Carbohydrate: 36 g

Cholesterol: 68 mg

Sodium: 896 mg

Sugar: 0 g

Fiber: 12 g

Squash Apple Bake Recipe

Weight Management & Bariatrics

SERVINGS: 6

INGREDIENTS

1 medium butternut squash, peeled and cut into 3/4 inch cubes

2 medium apples, peeled, cored, and cut into thin wedges

1 Tbsp Splenda

1 Tbsp all-purpose flour

1/4 cup melted butter

1/2 tsp salt

2 tsp ground cinnamon

DIRECTIONS

1. Mix squash and apples together in a casserole dish.

2. Blend other components and spoon over apples and skillet and blend together.

3. Bake, Covered, at 350 degrees F for 50 -- 60 minutes, or till tender.

4. Should you Such as a crispier topping, take off lid casserole dish for last 10 minutes of ingestion

NUTRITIONAL ANALYSIS PER SERVING (⅙ of a pan)

Calories: 133

Fat: 8 grams

Protein: 1 gram

Carbohydrate: 17 g

Cholesterol: 20 mg

Sodium: 445 mg

Sugar: 8.3 gram

Protein Packed Pesto Recipe

Weight Management & Bariatrics

SERVINGS: 4

INGREDIENTS

1/2 cup water

10oz package frozen, chopped spinach (thawed and well drained)

1/3 cup 1% cottage cheese

1/3 cup fresh basil (or 2 Tbsp dried ginger) - refreshing Favored

2 Tbsp grated parmesan cheese

1 Tbsp olive oil

2 tsp garlic, minced

DIRECTIONS

1. Blend all ingredients in blender or food processor

2. Blend or Process until smooth

3. Spoon 1/2 Cup of mix on fish or poultry

NUTRITIONAL ANALYSIS PER SERVING (1/2 cup)

Calories: 77

Fat: 5 g

Protein: 6 g

Carbohydrate: 4 g

Cholesterol: 3 mg

Sodium: 292 mg

Sugar: 1 g

Tzatziki Greek Yogurt and Cucumber Sauce Recipe

Weight Management & Bariatrics

SERVINGS: 8-9

INGREDIENTS

3 cups fat-free plain Greek yogurt

3 Tbsp lemon juice

1 garlic clove, chopped

2 medium cucumbers, peeled, seeded & diced

1 Tbsp salt

1 Tbsp finely chopped dill

Salt & pepper to taste

DIRECTIONS

1. Peel cucumbers and cut in half lengthwise. Simply take a little spoon and scrape out and discard the seeds.

2. Dice Cucumbers and place them in a colander with 1 Tbsp salt. Let stand for 30 minutes to draw the water out. Drain well and wipe dry cucumber bits with paper towel.

3. In a food Chip using a metal blade, include garlic, peppermint, lemon juice, dill, and several grinds of black pepper.

4. Procedure Until well mixed.

5. Stir the Mix to the yogurt.

6. Taste Before adding any excess salt, then salt if necessary.

7. Set in Refrigerator for two hours before serving so flavors can combine (don't detract from the resting time!!!) .

8. Drain off Any surplus water and stir before serving.

NUTRITIONAL ANALYSIS PER SERVING (1 cup)

Calories: 53

Fat: 0 g

Protein: 6 g

Carbohydrate: 8 g

Cholesterol: 1.7 mg

Sodium: 839 mg

Sugar: 7 g

Fiber: 0.3 g

Fantastic Morning Casserole Recipe

Weight Management & Bariatrics

SERVINGS: 4

INGREDIENTS

4 pieces of bread, crust trimmed

11/2 cups of egg replacement

11/2 cups skim milk

4 slices cooked turkey bacon, crumbled

1/4 cup (1 oz) shredded reduced-fat cheddar cheese

1/4 cup (1 oz) shredded reduced-fat Swiss cheese

1/2 cup chopped mushrooms

1/4 tsp seasoned salt

1/2 cup frozen hash brown potatoes, thawed

DIRECTIONS

1. Around bottom of lightly greased 9x9 inch baking dish, arrange bread slices, slightly overlapping. Put aside.

2. In big Bowl, beat together egg substitute, milk, turkey bacon, two Tablespoons all cheddar and Swiss cheeses, mushrooms, and salt.

3. Pour Mixture over bread pieces

4. Sprinkle Potatoes and remaining cheese over egg mix.

5. Cover and refrigerate overnight.

6. Bake, Discovered, in pre-heated 350 degree F oven until lightly browned and knife inserted near center comes out clean (about 40-45 minutes).

NUTRITIONAL ANALYSIS PER SERVING (1/4 pan)

Calories: 253

Fat: 8 g

Protein: 22 g

Carbohydrate: 22 g

Cholesterol: 18 mg

Sodium: 674 mg

Sugar: 7 g

Fiber: 2 g

Cool Ranch Veggie Pizza Recipe

Weight Management & Bariatrics

SERVINGS: 8

INGREDIENTS

Two LaTortilla Factory (or other comparable) low-carb wraps (big)

1/2 cup reduced fat chive and onion cream cheese

1/2 cup light sour cream

1 package Hidden Valley Ranch Dressing (use dry mixture)

⅛ cup shredded carrots

3/4 cup uncooked broccoli

3/4 cup diced tomatoes

⅛ cup diced green pepper

⅛ cup diced cucumbers

3/4 cup Kraft Light shredded Colby & Monterey Jack cheese

1/2 cup chopped black olives

DIRECTIONS

1. Mix cream Cheese, sour cream, and ranch dressing package together.

2. Spread evenly on tortillas.

3. Top with Veggies and olives and scatter.

4. Cut each tortilla into four pieces and serve.

NUTRITIONAL ANALYSIS PER SERVING (1/4 Tortilla)

Calories: 170

Fat: 10 g

Protein: 10 g

Carbohydrate: 12 g

Cholesterol: 23 mg

Sodium: 870 mg

Sugar: 1.6 g

Fiber: 4 g

Creamy Pumpkin Mousse Recipe

Weight Management & Bariatrics

SERVINGS: 4

INGREDIENTS

1 15-ounce cans pumpkin

1 4-ounce bundle skillet vanilla batter

2 cups sugar-free whipped topping (i.e., Cool Whip)

1/2 cup skim milk

1 teaspoon cinnamon

Allspice, nutmeg, ginger, clove and Splenda, to taste

DIRECTIONS

1. Mix all Ingredients together.

2. Whip until creamy smooth.

NUTRITIONAL ANALYSIS PER SERVING (1 cup)

Calories: 149

Fat: 4.4 g

Protein: 2 g

Carbohydrate: 28 g

Cholesterol: 0 milligrams

Sodium: 71 mg

Sugar: 8.6 g

Fiber: 3.4 g

Easy Chicken Tetrazzini Recipe

Weight Management & Bariatrics

SERVINGS: 6

INGREDIENTS

1 Tbsp. reduced-calorie margarine

1/2 cup scallions, sliced (approximately 5 scallions)

8 oz button mushrooms, sliced

3 Tbsp. all-purpose flour

1/4 tsp. Garlic powder

1/8 tsp. Black pepper

1 cup grilled chicken broth

1/2 cup fat-free skim milk

1/2 cm cooked, boneless, skinless chicken breasts, cubed

1/4 cup roasted pimentos, drained and chopped (roughly equal to a 2 oz jar)

2 Tbsp. sherry cooking wine

31/2 Tbsp. grated parmesan cheese

8 oz uncooked spaghetti, broken into thirds and cooked

DIRECTIONS

1. Melt Margarine in a large saucepan over medium-high warmth. Add scallions and mushrooms and cook till tender, stirring, about 5 minutes

2. Blend flour, garlic powder, pepper, broth, and milk in small bowl. Mix until well mixed.

3. Add flour mixture to saucepan. Cook until mixture boils and thicken, stirring constantly, for about ten minutes.

4. Insert Poultry, pimentos, and sherry. Cook until thoroughly heated, stirring occasionally, for approximately 2 minutes.

5. Stir in cheese and cooked spaghetti and toss gently.

NUTRITIONAL ANALYSIS PER SERVING (approximately 1 cup)

Calories: 167

Fat: 3 g

Protein: 10 g

Carbohydrate: 25 g

Cholesterol: 30 mg

Sodium: 175 mg

Sugar: 1.5 g

Fluffy Jello Recipe

Weight Management & Bariatrics

SERVINGS: 4

INGREDIENTS

1 box sugar jello, any taste

8 T. of Cool Whip Free

DIRECTIONS

1. Make jello according to directions on box

2. Place in Refrigerator to place

3. Once defined, Split jello to four 1/2 cup portions

4. Vigorously Blend 2 T. of Cool Whip Free with every 1/2 cup

serving

NUTRITIONAL ANALYSIS PER SERVING (half a cup)

Calories: 30

Fat: 0 g

Protein: 1 g

Carbohydrate: 2 g

Cholesterol: 0 milligrams

Sodium: 65 mg

Sugar: <1 g

Stuffed French toast Recipe

Weight Management & Bariatrics

SERVINGS: 1)

INGREDIENTS

4 Slices reduced calorie bread (35kcal per piece)

1/2 cup fat-free ricotta cheese

2 packets sugar substitute

3 egg whites

Dash of Salt

1/4 tsp pumpkin pie spice

Dash of Vanilla

Cooking spray

DIRECTIONS

1. Split Ricotta evenly between two pieces of bread.

2. Sprinkle 1 packet of sugar replacement on every slice of bread.

3. Place Remaining bread on top, which makes two sandwiches.

4. Beat egg whites. Add a dash of salt and 1/4 tsp pumpkin pie spice and a dash of vanilla to egg whites and stir fry.

5. Dip Sandwiches in egg whites and fry in skillet with small quantity of cooking spray.

6. Brown on Either side.

NUTRITIONAL ANALYSIS

Calories: 227

Fat:.5 g

Protein: 25 g

Carbohydrate: 27 g

Cholesterol: 20 mg

Sodium: 659 mg

Sugar: 8 g

Sweet and Sour Pork Recipe

Weight Management & Bariatrics

SERVINGS: 6

INGREDIENTS

Cooking spray

1 lb lean pork tenderloin, cut into thin strips

15 oz canned, unsweetened pineapple chunks

1/2 cup water

1/4 cup Splenda brown sugar mix

2 Tbsp corn starch

1/2 teaspoon table salt

1 Tbsp low-sodium soy sauce

2 medium green peppers, sliced (as tolerated)

1 small onion, sliced (as tolerated)

3 cups cooked brown rice

1/3 cup wine vinegar

DIRECTIONS

1. Heat a Nonstick skillet coated with cooking spray on medium-high warmth.

2. Add pork and cook till golden brown. Remove from skillet and set aside. Drain any residual fat from skillet.

3. Drain Pineapple chunks, reserving juiceset aside.

4. Blend Water, sugar, vinegar, cornstarch, salt, soy sauce, and reserved lemon juice in a small bowl. Add to skillet and cook until sauce is thickened, about two minutes.

5. Add pork To skillet and cook on low heat till meat is tender, stirring occasionally, for approximately half an hour.

6. Insert Celery, onion, celery, and pineapple chunks and cook for another five minutes.

7. Drink Over rice.

NUTRITIONAL ANALYSIS PER SERVING (1 cup of pork mix and 1/2 cup of rice)

Calories: 248

Fat: 3.5 g

Protein: 18 g

Carbohydrate: 36 g

Cholesterol: 60 mg

Sodium: 354 mg

Sugar: 8 g

Turkey Bean Enchilada Recipe

Weight Management & Bariatrics

SERVINGS: 4

INGREDIENTS

6 medium scallions, green and white parts chopped

2 cups cooked legumes, white turkey meat, cubed

15 oz canned pinto beans, drained and rinsed

1 cup canned enchilada sauce or taco sauce, divided

4 medium-sized fat-free or low-fat tortillas

1/2 cup shredded reduced fat Mexican cheese

DIRECTIONS

1. Preheat Oven to 350 degrees.

2. Blend scallions, turkey, beans, and 1/2 cup enchilada or taco sauce.

3. Fill each Tortilla using 1/4 of turkey-bean mix. Fold in sides, top and bottom of tortilla to completely enclose filling.

4. Place tortillas seam side down in a 9x13 inch baking dish.

5. Pour Staying 1/2 cup of sauce on the top of enchiladas and top with cheese.

6. Cover pan and bake until heated through and cheese is hot and bubbly (about 20 minutes)

NUTRITIONAL ANALYSIS PER SERVING (1 ENCHILADA)

Calories: 175

Fat: 3 g

Protein: 14 g

Carbohydrate: 19 g

Cholesterol: 27 mg

Sodium: 815 mg

Sugar: 3 g

Turkey Turnover Recipe

Weight Management & Bariatrics

SERVINGS: 24

INGREDIENTS

1 envelope dry onion soup

1 lb ground turkey (breast feeding only)

1 cup shredded 2% low fat

3 capsules decreased fat refrigerated crescent rolls (8 each Tubing)

DIRECTIONS

1. Preheat Oven to 350 degrees

2. Mix soup With beef in skillet and brown nicely

3. Blend in cheese

4. Unroll Dough, different rolls, and cut each triangle in half

5. Place Spoonful of beef mixture in center of each triangle

6. Twist Over, seal edges, and put on cookie sheet

7. Bake for 15 minutes

NUTRITIONAL ANALYSIS (two TURNOVERS)

Calories: 155

Fat: 7 g

Protein: 9 g

Carbohydrate: 13 g

Cholesterol: 14 mg

Sodium: 472 mg

Sugar: 3 g

Whopper Veggie Burger Recipe

Weight Management & Bariatrics

SERVINGS: 1)

INGREDIENTS

1 Boca Burger (Savory Mushroom Mozzarella taste; located in grocer's Freezer)

1 whole wheat hamburger bun (Healthy Life)

1 Tablespoon Light Miracle Whip

1 Tablespoon ketchup

1 Tablespoon mustard

Lettuce

Tomato

Onion

DIRECTIONS

1. Prepare Boca Burger as directed on package.

2. Place Hamburger on bun with mild miracle whip, ketchup, lettuce, onion and tomato.

NUTRITIONAL ANALYSIS PER SERVING

Calories: 260

Fat: 5.5 g

Protein: 18 g

Carbohydrate: 40 g

Cholesterol: 5 milligrams

Sodium: 1000 mg

Sugar: 9 g

You may also make this using really lean (95 percent) ground turkey Breast or very lean ground beef.

Bean Spread Recipe

Weight Management & Bariatrics

SERVINGS: 2

INGREDIENTS

1 can (15 ounce) canned pinto or kidney beans

Juice of 1 lime

Green or Red Tabasco sauce, to taste

Salt (optional)

DIRECTIONS

1. Mix all Ingredients together and combine with hand mixer or food processor

NUTRITIONAL ANALYSIS PER SERVING

Calories: 198

Fat: 1.5 g

Protein: 11.5 g

Carbohydrate: 34.5 g

Cholesterol: 0 milligrams

Sodium: 625 g

Sugar: 5 g

Balsamic Dijon Mustard Dressing Recipe

Weight Management & Bariatrics

SERVINGS: 4

INGREDIENTS

2 tbsp Dijon or whole mustard

4 tbsp balsamic vinegar

Pinch of oregano and pepper to taste

DIRECTIONS

1. Blend all ingredients

2. Insert Extra vinegar to flavor

NUTRITIONAL ANALYSIS PER SERVING (11/2 tsp)

Calories: 85

Fat: 0 g

Protein: 0 g

Carbohydrate: 26 g

Cholesterol: 0 milligrams

Sodium: 51 mg

Sugar: 0 g

Try out this flavored-packed sauce on leafy veggies, Poultry and poultry.

Light Alfredo Sauce Recipe

Weight Management & Bariatrics

SERVINGS: 8

INGREDIENTS

1 Tbsp. extra virgin olive oil

4 cloves garlic, minced

2 cups skim milk

1 cup chicken broth, heated

3 Tbsp. all-purpose flour

1/2 tsp. salt

1/4 tsp. Black pepper

1/2 cup grated Parmesan cheese

DIRECTIONS

1. In a Medium saucepan, heat olive oil on moderate heat.

2. Insert Garlic and sauté until aromatic.

3. Add flour And blend well until thick paste is formed.

4. Gradually Whisk in heated chicken broth.

5. Add milk, Salt and pepper.

6. Cook over Low heat until thick and smooth.

7. Stir in Parmesan cheese to complete.

NUTRITIONAL ANALYSIS PER SERVING

Serving size: 1/4 cup sauce

Calories: 71

Fat: 4 g

Carbohydrate: 5 g

Sugar: 3 g

Protein: 5 g

Serving suggestion: Serve over pasta or as a garnish for cooked boneless, skinless chicken breast, salmon or other fish.

Chicken Casserole Recipe

Weight Management & Bariatrics

SERVINGS: 4

INGREDIENTS

1/2 cup whole wheat pasta, raw (or 1 cup cooked)

1 cup cubed, cooked skinless chicken breast

2 cups frozen mixed veggies

1 can (10.5 oz.) 98% coconut lotion of chicken soup

1 cup 2 percent milk decreased fat shredded cheddar cheese

4 ounces. Canned mushrooms

3/4 cup water

Pepper, garlic powder and onion powder to taste

DIRECTIONS

1. Preheat Oven to 350 degrees.

2. Spray a 9x13 casserole dish with cooking spray.

3. Cook Pasta and veggies as directed on packages.

4. In a Large bowl, combine soup, poultry, 1/2 cup milk, cheese, mushrooms, water, cooked pasta and veggies.

5. Insert pepper, garlic powder and onion powder to taste.

6. Pour Mix into greased casserole dish, and sprinkle reserved cheese on top.

7. Bake Casserole until cheese is golden brown and tender, about 25-30 minutes.

NUTRITIONAL ANALYSIS PER SERVING

One serving = 1 cup of casserole

Calories: 256

Fat: 8 g

Protein: 19 g

Carbohydrate: 27 g

Sodium: 834 mg

Sugar: 3 g

Broccoli Egg and Cheese Bake Recipe

Weight Management & Bariatrics

SERVINGS: 8

INGREDIENTS

6 large eggs

4 oz light margarine

1/2 pound low-fat cheddar cheese

6 tbsp flour

2 pounds nonfat cottage cheese

10 oz frozen, chopped broccoli (thawed)

1 tsp salt

1 dash black pepper

1 dash paprika (optional)

4 ounce jar chopped pimento (optional)

1/2 cup chopped mushrooms, canned or fresh (optional)

DIRECTIONS

1. Preheat Oven to 350 degrees.

2. Blend all ingredients.

3. Spray 2-quart casserole dish with cooking spray.

4. Place Combined ingredients in pan and bake for 90 minutes.

5. Drink hot.

NUTRITIONAL ANALYSIS PER SERVING

Calories: 115

Fat: 5 g

Protein: 12 g

Carbohydrate: 5 g

Cholesterol: 75 mg

Sodium: 419 mg

Sugar: 2 g

Stuffed Cabbage Rolls Recipe

Weight Management & Bariatrics

SERVINGS: 6

INGREDIENTS

1 head of cabbage, person leaves removed

1/3 cup brown Minute Rice, or other whole grain of choice

1 tsp olive oil

1/2 medium onion, diced (if taken)

2 medium carrots, diced

1 pound 93% lean ground turkey

2 tsp garlic powder

2 tsp Oregano or Italian Taste

2 cups tomato sauce

DIRECTIONS

1. Preheat Oven to 350°.

2. Wash and Blanch* cabbage leaves for 30 minutes to create leaves easier to use.

3. Prepare rice as directed on package.

4. Meanwhile, At a large skillet, heat olive oil over moderate heat. Add the carrots and onions, stirring until slightly supple and soft.

5. Insert Turkey into the vegetables in skillet and cook till browned.

6. Insert the Powders and seasonings.

7. Blend Meat and rice.

8. Place 1/2 Cup of mixture into centre of 1 egg foliage. Roll up, sealing both ends as you roll.

9. Place Cabbage rolls in baking dish seam side downside by side to stop them from unrolling.

10. Top the Cabbage rolls with all the tomato sauce, allowing it to spill over towards the base of the dish.

11. Bake for 35-45 minutes. Let stand for 5-10 minutes before serving.

NUTRITIONAL ANALYSIS PER SERVING (1 roll)

Calories: 174

Fat: 5.5 g

Protein: 15 g

Carbohydrate: 16 g

Cholesterol: 54 mg

Sodium: 560 mg

Sugar: 6 g

*Blanching is a cooking technique where food is temporarily
Launched in boiling water (generally for 10-60 minutes).

Tuna Salad Recipe

Weight Management & Bariatrics

INGREDIENTS

1 can (6 ounce) Foods packed in water, drained

1 Tbsp. pickle juice

11/2 Tbsp. mayonnaise

1 Tbsp. powdered eggs

DIRECTIONS

Blend ingredients in a blender and puree until smooth.

NUTRITIONAL ANALYSIS PER SERVING

Serving size: 1/4 cup

Protein: 10 g

BBQ Roasted Salmon Recipe

Weight Management & Bariatrics

SERVINGS: 4

INGREDIENTS

1/4 cup lemon juice

2 tbsp fresh lemon juice

4 salmon fillets (6 oz each)

2 tbsp brown sugar

4 tsp chili powder

2 tsp grated lemon rind

3/4 teaspoon ground cumin

1/2 tsp salt

1/4 tsp cinnamon

DIRECTIONS

1. Preheat Oven to 400 degrees.

2. Blend First 3 components in Ziploc bag. Marinate in fridge for one hour, turning occasionally. Remove salmon from bag and discard marinade.

3. Blend Rest of ingredients and rub over fish. Put fillets in baking dish coated with cooking spray. Bake for 12-15 minutes until desired doneness. Drink lemon slice pops.

NUTRITIONAL ANALYSIS PER SERVING

Calories: 225

Fat: 6 g

Protein: 34 g

Carbohydrate: 7 g

Cholesterol: 88 mg

Sodium: 407 mg

Sugar: 6 g

Magically Moist Chicken Recipe

Weight Management & Bariatrics

SERVINGS: 12

INGREDIENTS

3 pounds skinless, boneless chicken breasts

11/4 cups whole wheat Italian bread crumbs

1/2 Smart Balance Omega plus Light Mayonnaise Dressing (or other mild mayo of choice)

DIRECTIONS

1. Preheat Oven to 425°.

2. Brush Mayonnaise on poultry.

3. Pour Bread crumbs on a large plate and roll chicken till coated.

4. Place Chicken breasts at foil-lined pan and bake for 40-45

minutes or till meat thermometer registers 165°F.

NUTRITIONAL ANALYSIS PER SERVING

Calories: 233

Fat: 5 g

Protein: 37 g

Carbohydrate: 8 g

Cholesterol: 8 g

Sodium: 268 mg

Sugar: 0 g

Lemon Broiled Orange Roughy Recipe

Weight Management & Bariatrics

SERVINGS: 4

INGREDIENTS

3 tbsp lemon juice

1 tbsp Dijon mustard

1 tbsp olive oil

1/4 tsp ground pepper

16 ounce orange roughy fillets (4 oz each)

8 moderate lemon wedges

DIRECTIONS

1. Cover the rack of a broiler pan or a baking sheet with tin foil and spray foil with cooking spray.

2. Blend Lemon juice, olive, olive oil and ground pepper, stirring well.

3. Place Fish fillets on rack or baking sheet.

4. Brush Fillets with half of the lemon juice mixture, reserving the remaining half.

5. Broil Fish for 5 minutes or till fish flakes easily.

6. Drizzle the allowed lemon juice mixture over the fillets and add pepper to taste. Serve with lemon wedges.

NUTRITIONAL ANALYSIS PER SERVING

Calories: 114

Fat: 4 g

Protein: 17 g

Carbohydrate: 3 g

Cholesterol: 23 mg

Sodium: 157 mg

Sugar: 0 mg

Spinach Frittata Recipe

Weight Management & Bariatrics

SERVINGS: 6

INGREDIENTS

2 tsp vegetable oil

1 medium onion, sliced (if taken)

1 package (10 ounce) frozen chopped spinach, thawed and drained

11/2 cups shredded reduced-fat cheddar cheese

4 egg whites

2 whole eggs

1/3 cup reduced-fat cottage cheese

1/4 tsp cayenne pepper

⅛ tsp salt

⅛ tsp nutmeg

DIRECTIONS

1. Heat oven to 375 degrees. Coat a 9-inch dish pan with vegetable oil spray.

2. In a Medium frying pan, heat oil on medium high. Add onion and cook 5 minutes until softened.

3. Insert Lettuce and cook 3 more minutes, set aside.

4. Sprinkle Cheese pan. Top with spinach/onion mix.

5. In a Medium bowl, whisk egg whites and whole eggs, cottage cheese, cayenne pepper, salt and nutmeg. Pour mixture into pie pan spinach and cheese.

6. Bake 30 to 35 minutes or until just set. Let stand 5 minutes.

7. Cut into wedges and serve.

NUTRITIONAL ANALYSIS PER SERVING (⅙)

Calories: 162

Fat: 8 grams

Cholesterol: 86 mg

Carbohydrates: 6g

Sugar: 0 g Protein: 16 g

Sodium: 548 mg

Crunchy Tuna Patty Recipe

Weight Management & Bariatrics

These crispy lettuce patties are excellent served with a squeeze of Lemon plus a dollop of fat-free Greek yogurt.

SERVINGS: 8

INGREDIENTS

4 3-ounce cans tuna, in water

4 egg whites

16 Wheat Thins crackers, crushed

1/4 cup grated carrot

1/4 cup sliced water chestnuts, capers or diced red pepper

1 Tbsp minced onion, if taken

Pepper, dill and dried mustard, to taste

DIRECTIONS

1. Mix all Ingredients together.

2. Form Mix into eight patties together with palms.

3. Spray Medium skillet with non stick cooking spray and set over moderate heat.

4. Cook patties Until golden brown on both sides, 2-3 minutes each side.

NUTRITIONAL ANALYSIS PER SERVING

Calories: 80 calories

Fat: 1 g

Protein: 12 g

Carbohydrate: 4 g

Cholesterol: 22 g

Sodium: 240 mg

Sugar: 0 g

Black Bean and Brown Rice Casserole Recipe

Weight Management & Bariatrics

SERVINGS: 8

INGREDIENTS

1/3 cup brown rice

1 cup vegetable broth

1 tbsp olive oil

1/3 cup diced onion

1 medium zucchini, thinly sliced

16 ounce cooked boneless, skinless chicken breast, breast into small pieces

1/2 cup chopped mushrooms

1/2 teaspoon cumin

1/4 tsp cayenne pepper

1 (15 ounce) can black beans, drained

1 (4 ounce) can diced green chilies

1/3 cup shredded carrots

2 cups low fat Swiss cheese, shredded

DIRECTIONS

1. Mix the Rice and vegetable broth in a pot, and bring to a boil. Reduce heat to low, cover, and simmer for 45 minutes or till rice is tender.

2. Preheat oven to 350? Degrees F.

3. Gently Dirt a large skillet with non cooking spray.

4. Heating Olive oil in skillet over moderate heat, cook onion until tender.

5. Mix in Zucchini, mushrooms, poultry, and seasonings.

6. Cook and Stir till zucchini is lightly browned and chicken is heated.

7. In big Bowl, combine cooked rice, onion, zucchini, mushrooms, poultry, beans, chilies, carrots, and 1 cup Swiss cheese.

8. Transfer to prepared casserole dish and sprinkle with remaining 1 cup Swiss cheese.

9. Cover Casserole loosely with foil, bake for half an hour in preheated oven.

10. Uncover, Continue baking 10 minutes until lightly browned.

NUTRITION FACTS

Serving size: 1/8 of recipe

Calories: 267

Total Fat: 6g

Total Carbohydrates: 22g

Dietary Fiber: 6g

Sugars: 1g

Protein: 31g

Spinach Frittata Recipe

Weight Management & Bariatrics

SERVINGS: 6

INGREDIENTS

2 tsp vegetable oil

1 medium onion, sliced (if taken)

1 package (10 ounce) frozen chopped spinach, thawed and drained

11/2 cups shredded reduced-fat cheddar cheese

4 egg whites

2 whole eggs

1/3 cup reduced-fat cottage cheese

1/4 tsp cayenne pepper

⅛ tsp salt

⅛ tsp nutmeg

DIRECTIONS

1. Heat oven to 375 degrees. Coat a 9-inch dish pan with vegetable oil spray.

2. In a Medium frying pan, heat oil on medium high. Add onion and cook 5 minutes until softened.

3. Add spinach And cook 3 more minutes, set aside.

4. Sprinkle Cheese in bowl. Top with spinach/onion mix.

5. In a Medium bowl, whisk egg whites and whole eggs, cottage cheese, cayenne pepper, salt and nutmeg. Pour mixture into pie pan spinach and cheese.

6. Bake 30 to 35 minutes or until just set. Let stand 5 minutes.

7. Cut into wedges and serve.

NUTRITIONAL ANALYSIS PER SERVING (⅙)

Calories: 162

Fat: 8 grams

Cholesterol: 86 mg

Carbohydrates: 6g

Sugar: 0 g Protein: 16 g

Sodium: 548 mg

Chapter 2 Gastric Sleeve Surgery basics guide

Vertical Sleeve Gastrectomy (Gastric Sleeve)

For a Lot of People, the gastric sleeve surgery in San Antonio, Texas is attractive because it isn't quite as extreme as a skip and it doesn't involve an implant such as the banding process. Together with the sleeve gastrectomy, there's not any dumping syndrome since there's not any re-routing of the intestines.

The perpendicular sleeve gastrectomy, also known as a"sleeve" or "gastric sleeve," is a hybrid vehicle operation. 80 percent of the gut is totally resected and taken out of the body. The resection is completed across the long axis of the gut so the new gut resembles a banana or a hockey-stick. The new gut is quite rigid, tubular and lean stomach, and doesn't enable you to eat very much food. The section of the gut that's eliminated is the very flexible.

With sleeve gastrectomy surgery, the weight loss results are Very much like bypass surgery for your first season or so. The process is generally covered by insurance.

Exactly why the vertical sleeve gastrectomy helps people Eliminate weight

The perpendicular sleeve gastrectomy is a metabolic surgery. By removing a part of the gut, we radically alter the neurohormonal pathways which control the feeling of appetite and how our body handles the calories we place in.

There's a hormone called ghrelin that's made primarily in The component of the gut that we eliminate. It's the principal driver in the appetite pathway, and with all the remarkable drops in ghrelin levels observed following the gastric sleeve surgery, we notice a commensurate drop in appetite! In addition, we see up-regulation of a hormone known as GLP1, which can be involved with all our body's management of sugar. In reality, many of the more recent diabetes therapy drugs are designed to up-regulate GLP1. The sleeve surgery does so without drugs and this manner; it can bring about remission of metabolic and cardiovascular disorder very quickly.

Benefits of sleeve gastrectomy surgery

Gastric sleeve weight reduction surgery Provides the next Benefits:

• May Reduce appetite, because less of this hunger-inducing hormone ghrelin is produced by your gut after the process

• Easier, Shorter operation compared to the usual gastric bypass (like a gastric bypass, gastric sleeve weight loss surgery does not re-route the intestines)

• No Adjustments are necessary, unlike with lap rings

• No Foreign items are left on your body

• Important Losing weight is the standard

• Weight Reduction is generally preserved

• No "dumping syndrome" with unpleasant side effects Which

Can Be associated with gastric bypass surgery

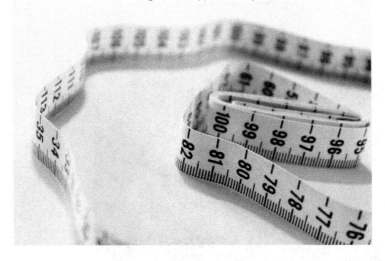

Who makes a fantastic candidate for gastric sleeve surgery?

These are important criteria that can help ascertain If you could be a fantastic candidate for gastric sleeve surgery:

BMI

Sleeve gastrectomy may be a Great option when you Have a body Mass index (BMI) of 40, which means that you're at least 100 pounds overweight. You could also qualify with a BMI of 35 in the event that you've got a chronic weight-related medical state, like type 2 diabetes, higher blood pressure or sleep apnea. Based upon your weight and BMI, you might be too hefty for gastric bypass surgery but nevertheless a fantastic candidate to get a gastric sleeve process.

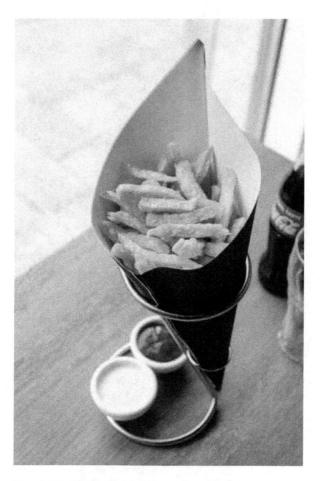

Total Wellbeing

If you are thinking about sleeve gastrectomy surgery, then you will Have weight-related wellness problems. But, you will have to have the ability to hold out against the physical strain of surgery. That is why we'll speak to you at length concerning your health history and present health, conducting some tests which may be necessary to make certain you're ready to physically take care of the surgery and healing.

Commitment to diet care

We'll make Certain you know your dietary principles and Assist you avoid eating more than you need to in the long run. Should you overeat, then it is likely to stretch your brand new, smaller stomach and recover weight. Our dietitians can help you adhere to a plan which meets your dietary needs and optimizes nourishment.

You will learn some very important tips, which you will need to follow rigorously. Some of the recommendations include:

• Chew everything well before consuming. Your dietitian can allow you to build this wholesome habit so you become a more aware eater until you've got the procedure.

• Eat Food and drink individually. You won't have a great deal of space in there. And additional liquid with food will make you feel full too quickly, which might prevent your ability to receive proper nutrition.

• Drink a Liquid 30 minutes prior to each meal. Hydration is also crucial to health. And before surgery, you truly get a great deal of liquid out of food you'll no longer have after surgery. So creating this wholesome habit guarantees that you get sufficient water to healthy kidneys, liver, liver and each component of the body.

• Prevent Calorie-packed foods and beverages that have little nutrient value. You are going to be eating less following the process, and therefore you want to make certain you've got space for healthy foods. That will not leave much space for anything else.

As an important aspect, some folks are moderators by Character and many others are abstainers. If you are a moderator, then you might be able to really occasionally and have junk food. However, and this is a big BUT: If you have problems moderating, as is true for the majority of individuals with the chronic illness obesity, then you are probably an abstainer. This means that you will be successful abstaining entirely because as soon as you get a preference, you've got difficulty stopping.

We frequently say "everything in moderation" However, this Philosophy does not work well for folks who have difficulty moderating. Should you have to abstain to become healthy, you have to make that commitment on your own. That frequently means never purchasing things you should not drink or eat. Simply keep them out of your property. You understand these methods pre-surgery to offer you the resources to maintain your commitment.

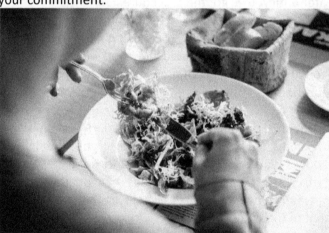

Commitment to exercise

Exercise is another important Part of your post-surgery Success. You ought to be happy to devote to exercising three or more times every week -- rather more. We've got a team of exercise physiologists that are especially trained to aid bariatric patients.

Willingness to take supplements that are nutritional supplements

Because you're brand new, smaller belly will maintain a much smaller Quantity of food; you are going to want to take multiple vitamin and mineral supplements for the rest of your life.

Emotional openness

Gastric sleeve surgery may have emotional consequences as well as physical ones. By way of instance, you might be employed to coping with stress from overeating, but if you do this following surgery, you can stretch your belly and recover the weight that you've worked so tough to lose. You could also see that some of your connections change. Bearing this in mind, we've got behavioral counselors on staff that will assist you navigate any emotional challenges you might face.

What's the gastric sleeve done?

The surgery can be completed in about one hour and can be minimally invasive. That is because BMI of Texas requires a laparoscopic approach to the process. As soon as you've gone to sleep because of general anesthesia, then your BMI surgeon makes several tiny incisions in your abdomen. Through these incisions, your physician inserts thin tubes. These home cameras and respective miniature surgical tools.

With this approach, your physician can definitely see what is happening inside without needing to open up you as with a typical open surgery. Your physician can create the surgical alterations to the gut safely and eliminate pieces of the gut, fretting about three-fourths of its initial mass during the tiny surgical incisions. This procedure reduces discoloration, surgical risks and healing time.

When the process is completed, the incisions will probably require a few stitches. Then you are prepared to enter recovery. What's gastric sleeve Recovery such as, you might wonder? Let us look at the second.

Things to expect post-op with gastric sleeve weight loss surgery

Using a sleeve, you need to expect to stay in the hospital to get A couple of nights. Your immediate targets after surgery would be to walk often and to do breathing exercises utilizing a special instrument called an incentive spirometer. Additionally, we'll provide you some blood-thinning medication to reduce blood clots. Patients are often permitted to start sipping liquids a few hours after surgery.

Post-op Day One aim: Transition entirely from IV fluids and drugs to oral ingestion and fluid pain medication. We utilize a distinctive three-day regional anesthetic at the very small incision websites so that the pain will be quite well-controlled.

Day 2: Many patients are ready to go home now. Do not feel bad if you aren't quite up for this. We realize that everybody differs, and we would like you to be entirely comfortable before we allow you to go home.

Post-Hospital Retrieval: After you leave the hospital you will be on a rigorous post-op regimen which will consist of intense limitations in what you may eat. But following one to two weeks you will re-establish the healthful eating and lifestyle habits you worked with your dietitian and other specialists since you ready for your surgery.

Which kind of weight loss may be anticipated?

Everyone differs, but people who've had gastric Sleeve surgery generally shed about 60 percent of the excess weight over 12 to 18 weeks. To put it differently, if you are 100 pounds overweight, you might shed 60 pounds over that time, but this amount could increase with appropriate diet and workout. In the mark, our patients have lost greater than average as a result of our own dietary, exercise and mental support.

How can be a gastric sleeve distinct in the gastric bypass?

In a gastric bypass, a surgeon makes a small pouch which bypasses the lower portion of your gut, sending food at the cap of the gut straight into the tiny intestines. The gastric sleeve is comparable, but the form and dimensions of the gut after the process is similar to that of a banana or hockey stick. This produces the practical gut more like a tube compared to a tote.

Gastric bypass could be harmful for People That have over 100 Pounds (45.36 kg)) To shed. In such scenarios, the gastric sleeve is significantly favored.

How do I prepare for my surgery date?

Leading up to the surgery date, you'll finish the Tests and instruction described previously. You will start practicing the skills you want to get a successful result. Exercise is significant since it requires some time to come up with a new habit. And in the event of a gastric sleeve process, your success is dependent upon your capacity to create new habits.

You can expect to eliminate some weight leading to the Process due to these changes. This shows your dedication to weight loss and maintenance success long term. The gastric sleeve surgery, in addition to the enormous support you get from our Texas staff, can help you become successful.

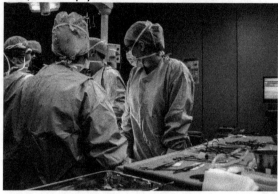

Two Weeks Pre-Op

In the 2 weeks prior to the surgery, you'll be on a really strict diet which helps shrink the liver and also prepare your body for a smooth transition to another means of living. An oversize liver would endanger your achievement and make the process more dangerous.

The pre-op diet normally includes calorie restriction as Well as low carbohydrates and massive quantities of lean protein.

Two Days Pre-Op

Two days prior to the process, your BMI of Texas physician will normally have you change into a liquid diet which might incorporate broth and protein shakes. You might also have the ability to drink decaf tea and coffee and consume Jell-O. However, your physician's orders may vary according to your special needs. You should avoid caffeine since this may affect your procedure.

Sleeve Gastrectomy Weight Loss Surgery

Sleeve gastrectomy patients can experience dramatic weight Reduction, but they have a lesser chance of developing a few of the complications related to gastric bypass. This surgery option doesn't reroute the intestinal tract.

This laparoscopic process is really a restrictive surgery that eliminates approximately 75% of their gut. Besides restricting the quantity of food a patient may eat, this decrease in gut size ends in the body making less of these hormones which stimulate hunger. Because of this, patients frequently experience long-term appetite suppression.

Through the sleeve gastrectomy process, a thin vertical Sleeve of gut is made with a stapling device. The sleeve-shaped gut remaining is more than the stomach pouch created throughout Roux-en-Y gastric bypass -- and is about the size of a banana.

Benefits

• Weight Loss. Sleeve gastrectomy patients shed 50 to 83 percent of the extra fat in the 12 to 24 months after surgery.

• Reduced Risks. Since the intestines aren't bypassed and the gut, though surgically reduced in size, functions normally, the danger of a few of the complications linked to gastric bypass is significantly decreased.

• Reduces Hunger Hormone. Since a substantial part of the stomach is removed, the creation of hormones in charge of sparking appetite is significantly reduced. Thus, patients feel full quicker using a significantly less quantity of food.

• Safer for High-risk Patients. Sleeve gastrectomy is an option for individuals with conditions that put them in an unacceptably large risk for different kinds of bariatric surgery.

Special Considerations and Risks

• Inadequate Weight Loss. Weight reduction might not be as quick or dramatic as for all those patients who have gastric bypass.

• Weight Gain. Patients may interfere with weight loss if they don't create the proper dietary modifications after surgery. Soft calories from foods like ice cream and milkshakes may be consumed and might slow weight loss.

• Leakage. This process requires the elimination of a part of the gut, and stapling generates the smaller stomach pouch. Complications can arise if a leak forms in the basic line. This acute postoperative issue is treated with antibiotics. Many instances cure with time. On the other hand, the leak could be severe enough to require urgent surgery.

• Not Reversible. Some of the stomach is permanently eliminated. Therefore, this Surgery can't be reversed, though it can be converted into gastric bypass and duodenal switch.

Conclusion

At a sleeve gastrectomy, also called a vertical sleeve gastrectomy or gastric sleeve process, the outer perimeter of the gut is removed to limit food consumption, leaving a sleeve of stomach, about the size and shape of a banana, and the pylorus, the muscle which regulates emptying of food from the stomach to the intestine. A sleeve gastrectomy is a purely restrictive procedure.

The sleeve gastrectomy, by reducing the size of their gut, allows the individual to feel full after eating less and taking in fewer calories. The surgery removes that part of the stomach that produces a hormone which can makes a person feel hungry.Sleeve gastrectomy is a much simpler operation than the gastric bypass process since it doesn't involve rerouting of reconnection of their intestines. The sleeve gastrectomy, unlike the Lap-band, does not call for the usage of a banding device to be implanted across some of the gut.

Contents

Introduction

Gastric Sleeve Surgery is now the hottest weight reduction operation on earth and causes significant and rapid weight reduction. Laparoscopic Sleeve Gastrectomy also referred to as the sleeve entails removing roughly 80 percent of their gut. The rest of the stomach is really a tubular pouch which looks like a banana. Gastric Sleeve surgery may be suitable weight reduction treatment for patients that aren't qualified for additional surgical procedures because of risk factors associated with a high BMI or other health conditions, including nausea. By abiding by the post-operative recommendations patients may expect to lose about 1 kilogram a week till their entire body weight reaches a healthful range. Because of a decrease in ghrelin, a hormone which affects appetite, patients will also be less inclined to feel hungry between meals. Restricts the total amount of food the stomach can hold - that the new stomach pouch carries a much smaller quantity than the standard gut and helps to significantly lower the total amount of food (and therefore calories) which may be consumed. The increased effect, but seems like the impact the surgery has on bowel tissues such as Ghrelin, the appetite hormone, which favourably suppresses appetite, reduces hunger, enhances satiety and enhances blood glucose control.gastric Sleeve surgery has a range of benefits over other weight loss processes. These are: Digestion works are preserved since the sole change is made to the dimensions of their gut.

Stomach nerves and openings remain intact and unaltered. The process for Gastric Sleeve surgery is laparoscopic, instead of open, meaning it's not as invasive, scarring will be minimal, and restoration will be faster.

As Gastric Sleeve surgery doesn't affect the digestive tract, healing times are somewhat faster than in other processes. Lower prospect of complications such as ulcers and other dangers related to gastric bypasses and lap-band surgeries. Involves a relatively short hospital stay of about 2 days When you have type 2 diabetes, evidence indicates that this ought to be a lot easier to control.

The disadvantages of Sleeve Gastrectomy will be the prospect of long term vitamin deficiencies, but this may be addressed by diet.

Chapter 1 what is gastric sleeve how it works?

CENTER FOR METABOLIC AND WEIGHT LOSS SURGERY
Sleeve gastrectomy is a surgical process that induces Weight loss by restricting food consumption. During this process, which is normally done laparoscopically, the surgeon removes about 75 percent of their gut. This ends in the gut taking on the form of a tube or "sleeve" that retains much less food. Although originally invented as the very first phase of a two phase process of superobese or high-risk sufferers, the sleeve gastrectomy is currently commonly and successfully used as a

destination process for weight loss in men with BMI over 40.

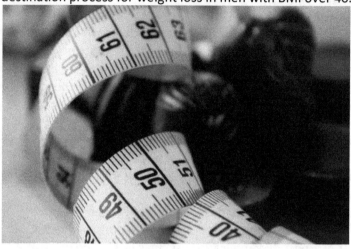

Gastric Sleeve

Statistically the documented weight loss with this particular process Ranges from 60 percent of their extra fat; better results are obtained with great adherence to dietary and behaviorial guidelines. With intelligent food choices, regular exercise and decent eating habits, individuals who've experienced a sleeve gastrectomy will appreciate and preserve decent weight reduction.

Together with the sleeve gastrectomy there's no foreign body Implanted, much like all the adjustable gastric band, and there's not any intricate intestinal rearrangement, much like all the gastric bypass. Many patients find that following a fair recovery, they are ready to comfortably eat a huge array of foods, such as meats and fibrous veggies. Contrary to the adjustable gastric band as well as also the gastric bypass, the sleeve gastrectomy is a permanent procedure -- it can't be reversed.

Removing some of the gut reduces the body's degree Of a hormone called ghrelin, which is often known as the "hunger hormone" Thus, a lot of men and women discover they are not as hungry following the sleeve gastrectomy. Ghrelin also plays a part in blood glucose metabolism, so individuals with type II diabetes often find an immediate decline in their need for diabetes drugs (particularly oral drugs) following the sleeve gastrectomy.

Advantages of Sleeve Gastrectomy

Sleeve gastrectomy induces rapid and effective weight loss much like gastric bypass surgery. Patients may expect to lose 50 percent or more of the extra weight in 3 years. The process doesn't require implantation of a ring, nor does this re-route the digestive procedure. Hormonal changes following the process assist patients to feel fuller eat, in addition to improve or solve diabetes.

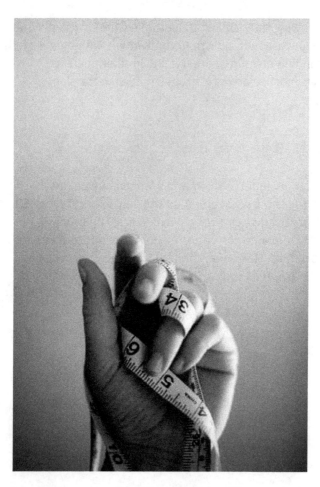

Disadvantages of Sleeve Gastrectomy

Like other surgical procedures, sleeve gastrectomy is non-reversible. The speed of premature surgical complications is similar to conventional gastric bypass. Patients are at risk for long term nutrient deficiencies.

What's Sleeve Gastrectomy Performed?

We do the sleeve gastrectomy as a laparoscopic procedure. This entails making five or six small incisions in the stomach and doing the process by means of a video camera (laparoscope) and lengthy tools that are put through these tiny incisions.

Throughout the laparoscopic sleeve gastrectomy (LSG), about 75 percent of the gut is removed leaving a lean gastric "tube" or "sleeve". No intestines have been removed or spilled through the sleeve gastrectomy. The LSG requires one or two hours to finish.

How Can Sleeve Gastrectomy Cause Weight Loss?

Sleeve gastrectomy is a restrictive process. It greatly reduces the size of your belly and restricts the total amount of food which may be consumed at any time. It doesn't cause decreased absorption of nourishment or bypass the own intestines. After eating a little bit of food, you'll feel full very fast and continue to feel full for many hours.

Sleeve gastrectomy can also lead to a reduction in appetite. In Addition to reducing the size of their gut, sleeve gastrectomy can lessen the sum of "hunger hormone" produced by the gut that might bring about weight loss following this process.

Who Would We Provide Laparoscopic Sleeve Gastrectomy?

This process is primarily used as part of a staged Strategy to surgical weight reduction. Patients that have a rather large body mass index (BMI) or who are at risk for undergoing a lengthier process because of lung or heart problems may benefit from the staged approach. Sometimes the choice to move ahead with a two-stage strategy is created before surgery because of such known risk factors. Quite simply, the choice to do sleeve gastrectomy (rather than gastric bypass) is created throughout the surgery. Reasons for creating this choice intraoperatively incorporate an overly big liver or scar tissue which would cause the gastric bypass process overly long or harmful.

In patients who experience LSG as a primary phase process, the Second phase (gastric bypass) is done 12 to 18 months after after substantial weight loss has happened and the possibility of anesthesia is a lot lower (and also the liver has diminished in size). Though this strategy involves two procedures, we think it's effective and safe for patients.

Laparoscopic sleeve gastrectomy may also be utilized as a Principal procedure. There's relatively little information concerning the use of LSG as a standalone process in patients with lower BMI's and it ought to be regarded as an investigational process in this patient category.

What Are The Dangers of Laparoscopic Sleeve Gastrectomy?

There are dangers that are typical to any laparoscopic Process like bleeding, infection, injury to other organs, or the requirement to convert to an open process. There's also a small risk of a flow from the basic line used to split the gut. These issues are infrequent and significant complications occur less than 1 percent of their time.

Overall, the operative risks associated with LSG are slightly greater than those found using the laparoscopic adjustable group but lower compared to the dangers related to gastric bypass.

What Are The Advantages Of Laparoscopic Sleeve Gastrectomy?

Based on their pre-operative weight, patients may expect to drop between 40% to 70 percent of the excess body fat in the first year following surgery.

Much obesity-related comorbidity improves or fix after bariatric surgery. Diabetes, hypertension, obstructive sleep apnea and abnormal cholesterol levels have been treated or improved in over 75 percent of patients experiencing LSG. Though long-term studies aren't yet accessible, the weight loss that happens after LSG contributes to remarkable improvement in those medical conditions from the first year following surgery.

Is Laparoscopic Sleeve Gastrectomy A Great Choice For Me?

Your physician may speak with you about LSG instead if you Have a BMI over 60 or important medical issues that increase your risk for getting anesthesia or gastric bypass. Laparoscopic sleeve gastrectomy might also be provided as part of a clinical evaluation when you've got a lower BMI and diabetes.

You should discuss all the available surgical procedures Together with your physician and decide which process is ideal for you.

Things to Know About Gastric Sleeve Weight Loss Surgery

1 approach to tackle obesity would be with regular surgery. This Kind of surgery involves removing or diminishing the size of your tummy. Bariatric surgery typically contributes to rapid weight reduction.

Gastric sleeve surgery is one of several Kinds of bariatric Surgery choices. Medical professionals typically call it vertical sleeve gastrectomy.

In this Guide, you'll have a closer look at what is involved in gastric sleeve surgery, such as its efficacy and potential complications.

What exactly does gastric sleeve surgery demand?

Gastric sleeve surgery is almost always performed as a invasive procedure using a laparoscope. This usually means a very long, thin tube is inserted into your abdomen through several tiny incisions. This tube has a light and a small camera attached to it and many tools.

Gastric sleeve surgery is performed with general anesthesia, which is medication that puts you right into a really deep sleep and takes a ventilator to breathe for you during the surgery.

The surgery involves dividing your gut into 2 unequal Components. Approximately 80 percent of those outer curved portion of your gut is cut off and removed.

The advantages of the remaining 20 percent are then stapled or sutured together. This produces a banana-shaped stomach that is just about 25% of its initial size.

You are going to be at the living room about one hour. After the Surgery is finished, you're going to be moved into the recovery area for health care. You are going to be at the recovery area for one more hour or so as you awaken from the anesthesia.

The tiny incisions in your abdomen typically cure fast. The minimally invasive nature of this surgery makes it possible to recuperate faster than a process where your stomach is started using a bigger incision.

Unless there are complications, you should have the Ability to go Home within two or three days following the surgery.

Is it successful?

Gastric sleeve surgery helps you Eliminate weight in two manners:

• Your Stomach is considerably smaller in order to feel full and stop eating earlier. As a result, that you take in fewer calories.

• The component of the stomach that generates ghrelin -- a hormone that is connected with appetite -- has been eliminated, which means you are much less hungry.

According to the American Society of Metabolic and Allergic Surgery, you can expect to lose at least 50 per cent of your extra weight over the 18 to 24 weeks after gastric sleeve surgery. Some people today lose 60 to 70 percent .

It is Important to Keep in Mind that this Is Only Going to happen if you Are dedicated to adhering to the diet and exercise plan recommended by the physician. By embracing these lifestyle modifications, you are more inclined to keep the weight off long term.

Weight reduction benefits

Losing a significant Number of excess weights can improve Your quality of life also make it less difficult to carry out many daily tasks.

Another important advantage of weight reduction is that the reduced risk Of obesity-related wellness conditions. These include:

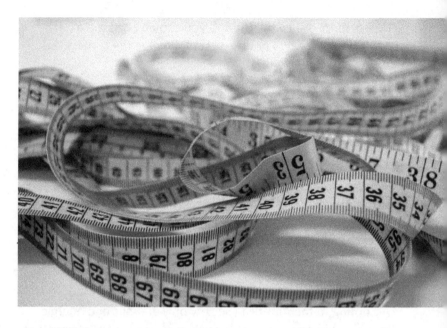

- Type 2 diabetes

- Significant cholesterol (hyperlipidemia)

- Significant Blood pressure (hypertension)

- Obstructive Sleep apnea

Who's a fantastic candidate for this surgery?

Bariatric surgery of any type, such as gastric sleeve Surgery, is just considered choice when powerful efforts to boost your diet and exercise habits, and also the usage of weight-loss drugs, have not worked.

Even after that, you have to meet specific standards to be eligible for a regular procedure. These standards are based on the own body mass index (BMI) and if you have some obesity-related wellness conditions.

Qualifying conditions:

• Intense (morbid) obesity (BMI rating of 40 or greater)

• Obesity (BMI rating of 35 to 39) with one important obesity-related condition

Sometimes, gastric sleeve surgery is completed if you are Obese but do not fulfill the standards for obesity, however, you get a substantial health condition associated with your weight.

What are the complications and risks?

Gastric sleeve surgery is known as a relatively safe procedure. But like all significant surgeries, there may be dangers and complications.

Some complications may happen after any surgery. All these include:

• Hemorrhage. Bleeding in your surgical wound or within your body may result in shock when it is intense.

• Deep vein thrombosis (DVT). Surgery as well as the healing procedure can boost your chance of a blood clot forming on your vein, usually in a leg vein.

• Pulmonary embolism. A pulmonary embolism can occur when a part of a blood clot breaks off and travels to your lungs.

• Irregular heartbeat. Surgery may boost the danger of an irregular pulse, particularly atrial fibrillation.

• Pneumonia. Pain can permit you to take shallow breaths that may result in a lung disease, such as pneumonia.

Gastric sleeve surgery may have added complications. A few possible side effects that are specific to this surgery include:

• Gastric leaks. Stomach fluids can flow in the suture line on your gut where it had been stitched back together.

• Stenosis. Section of your gastric sleeve may shut, resulting in an obstruction in your stomach.

• Vitamin deficiencies. The part of your gut that is eliminated is partially responsible for the absorption of vitamins that your body needs. If you don't take vitamin supplements, then this may result in deficiencies.

• Heartburn (GERD). Reshaping your gut can cause or aggravate heartburn. This may normally be treated with over-the-counter drugs.

It is Important to Keep in Mind that changing your diet and Exercise habits are crucial to losing the weight and keeping it off following gastric sleeve surgery. It is potential to gain the weight back if you

• eat also much

• consume an unhealthy diet

• exercise too little

Other concerns

Another Frequent concern, especially Once You Eliminate Lots of Weight fast, is that the massive number of surplus skin you might be left with as the pounds drop away. This is a frequent complication of gastric sleeve surgery.

This excess skin could be removed if it disturbs you. But remember it may take around 18 months for the body to stabilize following gastric sleeve surgery. That is why it's generally better to wait until considering a skin removal process. Until then, you might want to try out some strategies for tightening loose skin.

Another thing to think about before choosing to have gastric Sleeve surgery is that, unlike any other regular surgeries, gastric sleeve surgery is permanent. If you aren't satisfied with the outcome, your tummy cannot be transformed back to how it was.

How can your diet alter following gastric sleeve surgery?

Before gastric sleeve surgery is completed, you typically must consent to particular lifestyle modifications recommended by your physician. These changes are supposed to assist you reach and sustain weight loss.

One of these changes involves eating a healthy diet for the remainder of your life.

Your physician will recommend the very best gastric sleeve diet to get you after your surgery. The dietary modifications your surgeon proposes may be like the overall dietary guidelines under.

Dietary changes

• Two weeks Prior surgery. Boost protein, lower carbs, and remove sugar from the dietplan.

• Two days before and the first week following surgery. Ingest only clear fluids which are caffeine- and - carbonation-free.

• For the Next three months. It's possible to add pureed food into your dietplan.

You will usually have the Ability to eat regular, Wholesome food about 1 month following your surgery. You might discover that you just eat less than prior to the process since you will get full fast and will not feel overly hungry.

Your restricted diet and smaller foods may cause some Nutritional deficiencies. It is important to compensate for this by choosing multivitamins, calcium supplements, a monthly B-12 shot, and many others as recommended by your physician.

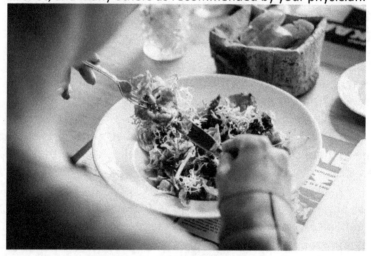

Is it covered by insurance?

In the USA, most health insurers realize that obesity is a risk factor for other health conditions that may result in serious medical issues. Because of this, many insurance businesses cover gastric sleeve surgery for those who have a qualifying state.

In accordance with the Centers of Medicare & Medicare Services (CMS), Medicare will cover gastric sleeve surgery if you meet the following requirements:

• Your BMI is 35 or greater

• You've one or more obesity-related health ailments

• You had been not able to eliminate the weight by simply modifying your diet and exercise habits or simply by taking drugs

Medicare does not cover gastric sleeve surgery in case you are Obese but do not possess an obesity-related health state.

Without health insurance policy, the price of gastric Sleeve surgery may vary widely from 1 area into another, and also from 1 centre to another in the exact same geographical location. Normally, the price could range from $15,000 to over $25,000.

Given this wide variation, it is Ideal to study and Speak to Several operative and surgeons facilities to find one you are comfortable with -- and also one which satisfies your budget.

The Main Point

Gastric sleeve surgery is one of several Kinds of bariatric Surgery choices. It works by making your stomach smaller so that you eat less. Since the dimensions of the gut are reduced, you will also realize that you are less hungry.

To be eligible for gastric sleeve surgery, you need to meet specific criteria. You have to show that you have attempted other weight-loss strategies -- such as diet, exercise, and weight loss medicines -- with no success. Other qualifying standards comprise your BMI and if you have some obesity-related wellness conditions.

Should you follow a healthy diet and exercise regimen frequently after gastric sleeve surgery, you could have the ability to shed more than 50 per cent of your extra fat within 24 weeks.

However, as with the Majority of surgical procedures, there's the danger of side effects and complications. If you are considering gastric sleeve surgery, speak to your physician about whether you are eligible for this process and if it is a secure solution for you.

Long-Term Infection after Gastric Sleeve Surgery

Gastric sleeve surgery, also called a sleeve gastrectomy, removes about 80 percent of their gut to promote weight reduction. Besides the dangers inherent with any surgery, gastric sleeve surgery could lead to a vast range of physical and psychological health issues. Those associated with weight and nourishment straight stem from how the staying, tube-like section of the stomach can only hold about 4 oz or 120 milliliters--a substantial reduction from its regular capability.1

Risks vs. Rewards

The remarkable decrease in belly size which results from Gastric sleeve surgery means you may only consume about half a cup at a time (at least initially). Since the quantity of food which may be consumed is limited, the amount calorie which may be obtained in is diminished. This is what contributes to weight reduction.

Gastric sleeve surgery is irreversible and May Lead to positive Health results for obese men and women who've fought with achieving and maintaining weight loss. And general, gastric sleeve is deemed secure when compared to other commonly performed surgeries.

Deaths from the procedure are rare, and if done by a qualified physician, the surgery has minimum complications. Nevertheless, when they do occur, complications may range from minor annoyances to important and possibly life-altering troubles.

Severe complications are those that occur shortly afterwards surgery. They include pain, bleeding, antastamotic flows (from the links between the intestines), and blood clots.2 the chronic issues detailed here are long-term, which means that they appear or persist six months following the onset of surgery.

Surgery is a tool, not a magic bullet. It requires you to follow release directions, limit food consumption, and adhere to the program supplied by your physician. It's likely to overeat and possess minimum weight reduction after surgery. It's also likely to have a severe complication either because of inadequate adherence for your post-surgical strategy or the surgery itself.

Gastric Sleeve vs. Bypass vs. Banding

There are various kinds of bariatric surgery, of which Gastric sleeve is merely one. There are lots of differences between these, and you need to examine each these options with your physician prior to deciding a process so you are able to guarantee that what you select would be the ideal alternative for you.

Listed below are two key long-term factors to keep in Head:

• A gastric sleeve is permanent. Contrary to the gastric band process --in which the ring that "cinches" the gut to split it into 2 components could be removed if There's a difficulty --that the portion of the gut eliminated with the sleeve process Can't Be substituted if there are issues or complications using digestion.

• You will not shed as much weight using a gastric sleeve. While individuals who have gastric bypass surgery generally shed weight and maintain a greater proportion of extra weight long term in comparison with people who have gastric sleeve surgery, skip can pose with it's own set of hard long-term troubles.

• Weight and Nutrition

• While the Goal of gastric sleeve surgery would be to encourage weight reduction, there's a possibility you can not shed as much as expected or that you shed weight, but get it back. What's more, while the decrease in food intake makes it possible to reduce calories, which also means that you're consuming fewer calories --that could cause deficiencies.

• Failure to eliminate

• That is a Serious problem in which the surgery is unsuccessful for weight reduction. The pouch might be too big, the individual may dismiss discharge directions, or a different issue could be found that prevents weight reduction.

• Regain

• From the First days following the surgery, the stomach pouch that remains is quite little and will hold approximately half a cup of food at the same time. With time, the pouch stretches and can accommodate larger quantities of food in a single sitting. This dilation allows bigger meals to be absorbed and may eventually lead to weight reduction weight or stopping reduction beginning

• Losing Weight after surgery simply to acquire all of back it normally starts in the next year following surgery, if it happens at all. Bariatric processes are a excellent tool for weight reduction, but if customs aren't altered and preserved, it's likely to acquire some or all the surplus weight again.

• Nutritional Shortfalls

• Unlike Many gastric bypass surgeries, patients that have a gastric sleeve process don't have any change in their capacity to consume nutrients in the gut. On the other hand, the remarkable drop in food intake may result in problems in taking in sufficient nourishment. Problems such as nausea and diarrhea may also lead to problems with consuming enough nutrients and calories too.

• In such Cases, a perfect whole-foods diet might not be sufficient to provide all the requirements of their human anatomy. Because malnutrition can be extremely severe, your physician may suggest using vitamin and mineral supplements, medicine, and other interventions to keep you long-term.6

• Food Intolerance

• One of The advantages of a gastric sleeve is the fact that all foods may be consumed after the process; other bariatric surgeries need you to avoid particular foods. But, that doesn't mean that the body will endure all kinds of foods.

• A 2018 Study discovered that food tolerance diminished after perpendicular sleeve gastrectomy, especially in regards to foods such as red meat, rice, pasta, and bread. The researchers noticed that this is probably because of the physiological and anatomical alterations in limiting the quantity of food that you can consume at the same time.7

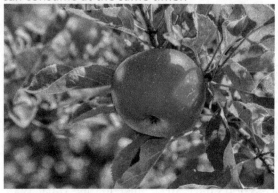

• **Physical Symptoms**

• Some Patients can experience gastrointestinal difficulties as a complication of gastric sleeve surgery. Although these may seem immediately after surgery, some patients might experience them for an elongated period of time. Sagging skin could be an additional complication which you experience after surgery.

• **Dyspepsia**

• Indigestion, Or an upset stomach, may be more regular following gastric sleeve surgery.8 this might be a result of the decreased volume of the gut and changes in how food goes through your gut and intestines.9

• Nausea

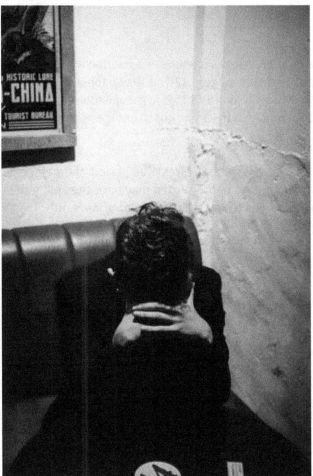

• Nausea is among the more prevalent issues that individuals face after sleeve gastrectomy.10 for many, this enhances after recovering from surgery, but for many others, the issue persists for weeks or long term.

• While it is not clear what causes nausea in this event, it can be partially as a result of food staying on your stomach for longer lengths of time.11 Nausea drugs can be found, which might be useful for many.

• Diarrhea

• For a few Patients, nausea is a severe issue that may persist following gastric sleeve surgery.12 This may happen for any range of reasons, such as alterations in gut microbiota and accelerated exposure to the small gut to undigested nutrients.13

• In instances Which last for an elongated period of time, the physician or even a gastroenterologist may have the ability to help stop nausea, which may result in malnutrition and dehydration.

• Signs You Are Dehydrated

• Sagging Skin Care

• This Complication is typical with all kinds of weight loss surgeries and can be caused by skin stretching throughout the time of obesity.14 A panniculectomy could possibly be an choice to get rid of extra skin, but many surgeons prefer to wait till the patient's weight has been steady for one or two years before removing extra skin.

• Medical Problems

• Gastric Sleeve surgery may cause medical conditions which range from moderate to severe. Speak to your physician if you have any worries about your probability of developing a health dilemma after surgery.

• **Persistence of Chronic Conditions**

• For a few, Eliminating chronic health problems--diabetes, hypertension, and many others --is your reason behind getting this surgery. Sometimes, these issues don't disappear after surgery, or else they might go away briefly from the first months or years following surgery and return afterwards.

• **Gastroesophageal Reflux Disease (GERD)**

• Heartburn, alongside other signs of GERD (bloating, feelings of fullness, and upset stomach), is common following this surgery and frequently requires medicine.5

• **Stomach Ulcers**

• Stomach Ulcers, called peptic ulcersare far somewhat more prevalent after gastric sleeve surgery And are generally diagnosed through an upper endoscopy following the patient Experiences bleeding (viewed as a dark, tarry feces or as blood in vomit) or pain In the gut region.

Gallstones

• Gallstones Are more prevalent following all kinds of bariatric surgery, building a cholecystectomy (surgery to remove the stomach) more prevalent to weight loss surgery patients.16

• **Stomach Obstruction**

• Scarring and narrowing of the outlet of the gut, also called stenosis, may make it hard or perhaps impossible to digest food. This complication is usually fixed by means of a physician that "stretches" or fixes the region which has been narrowed.

• **Abdominal Adhesions**

• The Organs and cells of the gut are obviously slippery, letting them slide past each other through movements like bending, twisting, and walking. After surgery, scarring may make these cells"stay" to each other. This induces a pulling sensation that can range from bothersome to debilitating with motion.Abdominal adhesions may also result in small bowel obstructions.

• **Abscess**

• An Abscess is a collection of infectious material (pus) that creates from the entire body in a pocket-like location. This typically happens shortly after the first surgery, because of spillage or leakage of intestinal contents. In the case of gastric sleeve surgery, abscesses have been diagnosed from the spleen, a few necessitating the manhood to be removed, but this Is Quite uncommon.

• **Delayed Leak**

• Most Suture line flows, also called suture line disruption or SLD, are found shortly after surgery. Sometimes, however, the region of the gut which was stitched together will start to flow months or years following surgery.

• These Later leaks are a lot milder but may be both annoying, and they might require drugs, hospitalization, or surgery to fix.

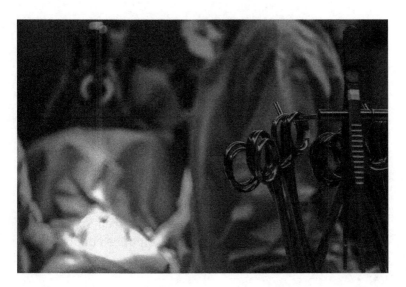

• Incisional Hernia

• A hernia can form at the website of any surgical incision. This danger is lessened by minimally invasive (laparoscopic) surgical methods, but a hernia may still form in the months and years after this type of process. Normally, that looks like a little bulge in the Website of a surgical incision.

• Psychological or Social Concerns

• Gastric Sleeve surgery can change your mental and psychological well-being, in addition to your relationships with other people. While weighing possible physical complications of this process is vital, these should not be overlooked.

• *Addiction Transfer*

• That is a Phenomenon that occurs to some people when they're not able to use food as a means to self-medicate their feelings. by way of instance, after a difficult day on the job, it's not feasible to go home and binge an whole container of ice cream--it simply won't match in the gut.

• Additional Kinds of addictions become more attractive since they're still possible using the smaller gut dimensions --alcohol misuse, drug abuse, and sexual dependency being one of the most frequent after surgery.

• Divorce

• From the United States, an average of 50 percent of marriages end in divorce; a few sources show that the speed of divorce following bariatric surgeries is as large as 80 percent.

• A 2018 Study indicated that divorce levels following gastric sleeve surgery might increase because the remarkable weight loss that impacts may impact the dynamics of a connection. This could occur if a spouse feels envious or no longer desired.

• Patients who are thinking of the surgery are advised to speak to their spouses about any possible problems and how they may handle anxieties should they appear.23 Couples might reap having this dialog with the assistance of a therapist.

• A Word by Very well

• One of The critical criteria that research scientists consider when assessing the success and security of operations is 10-year results. In cases like this, when it comes to the way patients maintain weight loss, what their general health resembles, and some other complications they've had because of surgery.

• It's Important to understand that gastric sleeve surgery is a fairly new process, so there's less 10-year information for gastric sleeve surgery than there is with other surgeries.

Therefore, more long-term complications may be added to the listing later on.

Chapter 2 Recipes You Need in Your Bariatric Life

Traditionally we find ourselves at one of Both of These ships:

• Tasty, But wicked OR

• Healthy, But not yummy

Try our choice: Delicious and wholesome

Have your bariatric foods left you frustrated? The dietary Restriction that accompanies being a patient could be troublesome to put it gently. Imagine if you did not need to sacrifice the foods you like or your weight loss progress?

At it's most elementary level, weight reduction is a statistics game. If We're frequently in a calorie excess (consuming more calories than our bodies burn off) we get weight, if we consume fewer calories than we burn off we lose weight. It is actually that easy. Why is it so tough to drop weight on a constant basis?

Successful meal prep and portion control fix this Issue altogether. If you'd like guilt-free, flavorful and portion-controlled foods that work at any meal program you want to try out those recipes!

Get precisely the nourishment you want, in the serving Sizes you will need

1 thing which Makes cooking in bulk or one-pot recipes (such as at a crockpot or a casserole) hard for meal-planning is that the amount of servings is not exact. Calculating the calories each serving necessitates busting a spreadsheet simply to receive your calories and macro amounts. Then you need to quantify out that quantity each time you get a serving. Not perfect.

Every recipe in this informative article yields individually packaged Single portions, making portion control as straightforward as it could be. It is possible to earn a whole batch and save the remainder for days and revel in stress-free, yummy meal-planning.

Chicken, Bacon and Ranch Wonton Cupcakes

This recipe brings All Your favorite tastes together in A tight, organized bundle. Who says you can not delight in the absolutely married taste of ranch and bacon when slimming down? Moderate ranch seasoning, bacon and lean chicken breast feeding make this an unbeatable alternative for healthier eating.

NUTRITION INFORMATION PER CUP:

152 calories | 10 g carbohydrates | 6 grams fat | 14 grams protein

INGREDIENTS

• 1 pounds uncooked boneless, skinless chicken breasts

• 1 Tbsp ranch seasoning

• two Tsp olive oil

• 5 pieces center-cut bacon, cooked crisp and chopped

- 3/4 cups Yogurt-based ranch dressing (like Bolthouse Farms)

- 24 wonton wrappers

- 4 ounces 2% shredded sharp cheddar

DIRECTIONS:

1. Preheat the oven to 375. Gently mist 12 cups at a normal muffin/cupcake tin with cooking spray and set aside.

2. Set the Raw chicken strips into a Ziploc bag and scatter with the ranch seasoning. Seal the bag and also shake/massage till the grain is coated with the seasoning.

3. Bring the Canola oil over moderate heat in a regular skillet. After the oil is hot, add the chicken pieces and stir them around to coat with oil. Arrange them into one layer and cook for 5-7 minutes, then turning sometimes, until the chicken pieces are cooked through. Remove the chicken to a cutting board and chop into small pieces.

4. Set the Chopped chicken into a mixing bowl and then stir in the chopped bacon and ranch dressing until well blended.

5. Push a Wonton wrapper to the base of all those coated cups in the muffin tin. With about half the chicken mixture, spoon evenly to the wonton wrappers. Sprinkle about half of the shredded cheddar evenly on the top of every cup. Press another wonton wrapper on top and repeat the layering steps together with the remaining chicken mixture and shredded cheddar.

6. Bake for 18-20 minutes before the wontons are golden brown and the materials are warmed through. Remove the muffin tin from the oven and allow cooling for 2-3 minutes before

removing from the tin

Sesame Chicken Wonton Cups

If Asian fusion at a crispy package is not enough to get you Excited then we've got a bigger problem on our handson. Chicken does not need to be dull and dull. Do not overlook the sesame seeds along with the cilantro to actually make this 1 stand out! Makes 24 Wonton Cups.

NUTRITION INFORMATION PER CUPCAKE:

152 calories | 10 g carbohydrates | 6 grams fat | 14 grams protein

INGREDIENTS

- 8 oz boneless, skinless chicken breast

- cooking spray

- 24 wonton Wrappers, about 6 ounces.

- two tablespoons tahini

- two tablespoons soy sauce or tamari sauce

- two tablespoons maple syrup

- two tablespoons mayonnaise

- 1/2 cup thinly sliced snow peas

- 1/2 cup shredded carrot

- 1/2 cup thinly sliced scallions

- two Tsp chopped ginger and/or cilantro

- Black sesame seeds for garnish, optional

DIRECTIONS:

1. Place Chicken breast in a skillet and cover with cold tap water. Place over high heat and bring to a simmer. Reduce heat to keep a gentle simmer and cook till the chicken is no longer pink at the middle and cooked through, 8 to 12 minutes, depending on the depth of the meat. Remove the chicken and let cool. Cut chicken into small cubes.

2. Meanwhile, preheat oven to 350°F. Coat two 12-cup mini-muffin tins with cooking spray. Cut off corners wonton wrappers to create an octagonal form. Gently press wrapper down into each cup. Lightly spritz wrappers with cooking spray.

3. Transfer the pans into the oven and bake till the wrappers have started to turn golden brown and so are crispy and simmer 10 to 14 minutes. Let cool completely.

4. Whisk Tahini, soy or tamari, maple syrup, and avocado in a medium bowl until smooth. Stir in the chicken and simmer until cold, 40 minutes to 1 hour.

5. Stir snow peas, carrots, scallions, and herbs into chicken mixture. Split the chicken salad one of wonton cups, about two litres tablespoons per day. Garnish with sesame seeds, if using. Drink immediately.

Meatloaf Muffin using Mashed Potato Frosting

While this can be another play around the cup-cake you have to give it the opportunity. If you prefer the basic principles of meatloaf and mashed potatoes you will enjoy every ideal snack of the healthful pairing. Use lean ground beef or turkey (at least 93% lean) and you're able to fit this to any diet. Makes 12 Cupcakes.

NUTRITION INFORMATION PER CUPCAKE:

120 calories | 12.25 g carbohydrates | 4.25 grams fat | 9 grams protein

INGREDIENTS

For your Meatloaf Cupcakes:

• 1.3 pounds 93% lean ground turkey

• 1 cup Grated zucchini, all moisture squeezed dry using a paper towel

• 2 tablespoon onion, minced

• 1/2 cup seasoned breadcrumbs

• 1/4 cup ketchup

• 1 egg

• 1 teaspoon kosher salt

For your Skinny Mashed Potato"Frosting":

- 1 pounds (about 2 medium) Yukon gold potatoes, peeled and cubed

- 2 big garlic cloves, peeled and halved

- 2 tablespoon fat-free sour cream

- 2 tablespoon Fat-free poultry broth

- 1 tablespoon skim milk

- 1/2 tablespoon Light butter

- Kosher Salt to taste

- Dash of Fresh ground pepper

- 2 tablespoon fresh thyme

DIRECTIONS:

1. Place the Garlic and celery in a large pot with salt and sufficient water to cover; contribute to a boil.

2. Cover and Decrease heat; simmer for 20 minutes or till potatoes are tender.

3. Drain and Pour onions and garlic into the pan. Add sour cream and remaining ingredients.

4. Employing a masher or blender, mash until smooth.

5. Season with pepper and salt to taste.

6. Meanwhile, preheat the oven to 350°.

7. Line a muffin tin with foil liners.

8. In a Large bowl, combine the turkey, zucchini, onion, breadcrumbs, ketchup, egg, and salt.

9. Place Meatloaf mixture into muffin tins, filling them to the surface, making certain they're flat in the top.

10. Bake Discovered for 18-20 minutes or till cooked through.

11. Eliminate Out of tins and put on a baking dish.

12. Pipe the "frosting" on the meatloaf cupcakes and function.

Chicken Broccoli Alfredo Wonton Cupcakes

If You want a healthy meal it generally will not contain Creamy Alfredo at any given capacity. Fortunately you are reading this recipe and will adore the way that it can fit into your diet if you're keeping your current weight or remain in your trip to your target weight. The Italian seasoning and light Alfredo sauce makes this feel like a cheat meal, you may return to the one many times! Makes 12 Cups.

NUTRITION INFORMATION PER CUP:

130 calories | 9 g carbohydrates | 5 grams fat | 13 grams protein

INGREDIENTS

- 1 1/2 Tsp olive oil

- 1 cup Broccoli florets, chopped little

- 2 cups cooked shredded or diced chicken breast

- 1 cup light Alfredo sauce

- 1/2 teaspoon Italian seasoning

- 1/8 Tsp black pepper

- 24 wonton wrappers

- 1 1/2 cup Shredded 2 percent Mozzarella cheese

- 1 Tbsp grated Parmesan cheese

DIRECTIONS:

1. Preheat the oven to 375. Gently mist 12 cups at a normal muffin/cupcake tin with cooking spray and set aside.

2. Pour the Oil to a skillet and deliver over moderate heat. Add the broccoli and cook for 5 minutes or until broccoli is tender, stirring occasionally.

3. Transfer the broccoli into a mixing bowl and blend with the chicken, alfredo sauce, Italian seasoning, and pepper. Stir until well blended.

4. Push a Wonton wrapper to the base of all those coated cups in the muffin tin. With about half the chicken mixture, spoon evenly to the wonton wrappers. Sprinkle about half of the

Mozzarella cheese evenly on the top of every cup. Press another wonton wrapper on the top and repeat the layering steps together with the remaining chicken mixture and Mozzarella cheese. After finish, sprinkle 1/4 tsp of Parmesan cheese on the top of each wonton cup.

5. Bake for 18-20 minutes until golden brown.

Skinny Meatloaf Muffins with BBQ Sauce

This is just in time for summer! No need to kick the bbq For great when choices like these yummy muffins are from the cards. Applying lean turkey or ground beef makes it a no-brainer for your own health-conscious along with also the foodie alike. Do not skimp on the Worcestershire sauce and then experimentation with different bbq sauces! Makes 9 Servings.

NUTRITION INFORMATION PER CUP:

115 calories | 18 g carbohydrates | 2 grams fat | 18 grams protein

INGREDIENTS

• 1 bundle (~1.25 lbs) 99 percent fat-free ground turkey breast

• 1/2 cup bread crumbs

• 1 cup onions, finely diced

• 1 egg

• two tablespoons Worcestershire sauce

- 1/2 cup barbecue

- 1/4 Tsp salt

- Fresh Ground pepper, to taste

DIRECTIONS:

1. Preheat Oven to 350 degrees. Coat a routine (12-cup) muffin pan with cooking spray. Because this recipe makes 9 meatloaf muffins, you will just fill 9, not 12. Put aside.

2. To create Bread crumbs: 1 piece or multigrain bread. Set in a blender and pulse before made into crumbs.

3. In a Large bowladd ground turkey, bread crumbs, onions, egg, Worcestershire sauce, 1/2 cup barbecue sauce, salt, and pepper. With your hands or a large spoon, then thoroughly blend together until well mixed.

4. Insert Meatloaf mix to the 9 muffin cups, flattening out the shirts. Top each meatloaf muffin using 3/4 tbsp skillet and spread evenly on top.

5. Bake for 40 minutes. Run a knife around each muffin to loosen it in the pan. Remove to a serving plate.

Crunchy Taco Cups

Mexican food is usually packed with cream, cheese and unnecessary fats. These generally calorie dense choices cause blissful overeating. If you create these taco cups you will find the best of both worlds: flavorful, south-of-the-boarder flavor without the guilt which normally follows! We enjoy low sodium taco seasoning. It tastes just as nice and it is ideal to prevent excessive sodium once we can. If you're feeling"elaborate," substitute the Rotel tomatoes with a few freshly grated tomatoes. The tomatoes and thin coating of melted cheese makes this an instant classic. Makes 12 Taco Cups.

NUTRITION INFORMATION PER CUP:

178 calories | 10.4 g carbohydrates | 7.3 grams fat | 16.8 grams protein

INGREDIENTS

• 1 pounds lean Ground beef, browned and drained

• 1 Envelope (3 tbsp) taco seasoning

• 1 (10-oz) can Ro-Tel Diced Tomatoes and Green Chiles

• 11/2 cups Sharp cheddar cheese, shredded (or Mexican mix)

• 24 wonton wrappers

DIRECTIONS:

1. Preheat Oven to 375 degrees F. Generously coat a normal size muffin tin with non stick cooking spray.

2. Blend cooked beef, taco seasoning, and berries in a bowl and stir to blend. Line each cup of the prepared muffin tin using a wonton wrapper. Insert 1.5 tsp taco mixture. Top with 1 tablespoon of cheese. Press down and put in a second layer of the wonton wrapper, taco mix, and a last layer of cheese.

3. Bake in 375 for 11-13 minutes before cups are warmed through and edges are gold.

Chicken Cordon Bleu Wonton Cupcakes

Chicken Cordon Bleu can make you think about a standard feast Hall buffet, however, give this a try and you will have a change of heart. 1 thing which Chicken Cordon Blue has gotten is that the mixture of cheese and flavorful noodle paired with lean, healthful chicken. Those aspects are not lost here in this ideal "cupcake." Makes 12 "Cupcakes.

NUTRITION INFORMATION PER CUP:

152 calories | 10 g carbohydrates | 4 grams fat | 17 grams protein

INGREDIENTS

• 12 ounce (two 1/2 cups) cooked diced or shredded chicken breast feeding

• 3 ounce thinly sliced deli ham, sliced

• 8 wedges Of the Laughing Cow Light Swiss Cheese Wedges, sliced

• 1 teaspoon mustard

• 24 wonton wrappers

• 6 pieces 2 percent Swiss cheese, each cut into 4 equal pieces

• 0.75 ounce seasoned croutons, crushed

DIRECTIONS:

1. Preheat The oven to 375. Gently mist 12 cups at a normal muffin/cupcake tin with cooking spray and set aside.

2. In a Microwave-safe mixing bowl combine the ham, chicken, chopped cheese wedges, and mustard and stir together. Set the bowl in the microwave and heat on high for 1 1/2 minutes till contents are still warm. Use a spoon to mix contents and smush the cheese wedges till they have coated the beef.

3. Push a Wonton wrapper to the base of all those coated cups in the muffin tin. With about half the chicken mixture, spoon evenly to the wonton wrappers. Put one of the two% Swiss bits on top of each cup. Press another wonton wrapper on the top and repeat the layering steps together with the remaining chicken mixture and 2% Swiss cheese.

4. Bake for 10 minutes and then remove it in the oven. Sprinkle crushed croutons evenly on top of each cup and then return the pan into the oven for another 8-10 minutes before the wontons are golden brown and the contents are warmed through.

Crab Salad at Crisp Wonton Cup

We Are in Need of variety in our diets, otherwise we get burnt out on Foods we might love and have loved for years! Chicken and steak are fantastic, but we want an offering from the sea to round out our diet. All these crab salad cups are exactly what you want if you are overlooking that flavor of the sea! Makes 18

"Cupcakes" (6 Servings) 1 Serving is 3 Cups!

NUTRITION INFORMATION PER CUP:

170 calories | 17 g carbohydrates | 7 grams fat | 9 grams protein

INGREDIENTS

For your Wonton Cups:

- Cooking spray

- 18 wonton wrappers

- two Tsp olive oil

- 1/4 Tsp salt

For the Dressing:

- 1 teaspoon lime zest

- two tablespoons fresh lime juice

- 1/4 Tsp salt

- 1/8 Tsp black pepper

- 1/2 teaspoon dried hot red pepper flakes

- two Tsp olive oil

For the Salad:

- 1/2 pound lump crabmeat

- 1 stalk Celery

- 1/2 cup finely diced mango

- 1/4 cup Thinly sliced scallions

- two tablespoons coarsely chopped fresh cilantro leaves

DIRECTIONS:

1. Preheat the oven to 375 degrees F. Spray two mini-muffin tins with cooking spray.

2. Brush the Wonton wrappers with acrylic, and then put each wrapper to a part of a mini-muffin tin. Gently press each wrapper to the tin and then arrange so that it creates a cup form. The wrapper will float itself and then stick up from this cup. Sprinkle with salt and bake for 8 to 10 minutes, until browned and crispy. Remove from the tin and permit wrappers to cool.

3. Meanwhile Whisk together the zest, lime juice, pepper, salt, and pepper flakes. Add the oil and whisk until well blended.

4. In a Medium bowl, toss together the crabmeat, cherry, celery, scallions, and cilantro. Add dressing and toss to blend. Fill each cup with all the crab salad and function.

Thai Chicken Salad Wonton Cups

Chicken salad could be as entertaining as waiting in the DMV, are we correct? Insert some Thai taste to this dull classic and you are really onto something. Chicken could be so versatile and that's evident in this yummy chicken salad cup. The wonton cup provides the essential pinch into the salad. The lime and citrus seeds actually provide this the different Thai taste you're certain to love. Makes 12 Cups.

NUTRITION INFORMATION PER CUP:

74 calories | 6.4 g carbohydrates | 2.4 grams fat | 6.2 grams protein

INGREDIENTS

- 12 wonton wrappers

Dressing:

- 1 garlic, smashed

- 11/2 tablespoon Lime juice

- 2 tsp rice vinegar

- Two 1/2 tsp Fish sauce

- 1 teaspoon soy Sauce

- 11/2 tablespoon Eucalyptus oil (or grapeseed, vegetable, or alternative neutral-flavored petroleum)

- 1 teaspoon sugar (or honey)

- 1 -- 2 Birds eye candy, deseeded and finely chopped (or 1 -- 2 teaspoon of chili paste or hot sauce)

Chicken Salad:

- 11/2 cups shredded cooked chicken

- 11/2 cups finely shredded cabbage

- 3/4 cup carrot, finely julienned

- 1/3 cup Finely chopped shallots/scallions

Garnish:

- Sesame seeds

- Fresh coriander/cilantro leaves

DIRECTIONS:

1. Preheat Oven to 160C/320F.

2. Place Wonton wrappers into a normal muffin tin, then molding it to the cups. Bake for 12 to 15 minutes, until crisp and pale golden brown. Remove from the oven and allow the cups cool from the muffin tin. Store in an airtight container until required (stays clear for as many as 3 times).

3. Blend Dressing ingredients in a jar and shake to blend. Put aside for at least 10 minutes to enable the flavors to infuse.

4. Blend Chicken Salad ingredients in a bowl and toss to blend.

5. To serve: Discard the garlic clove in the Dressing, and then chuck it via the Chicken Salad. Split the Chicken Salad between cups. Garnish with sesame seeds and cilantro/coriander, if using. Drink immediately.

Buffalo Chicken Cups

Are Buffalo wings wholesome? Obviously they're not. Can we Take pleasure in the flavor of buffalo wings and lose weight? Obviously we could. This recipe carries lean chicken and yummy buffalo sauce to make a multitude of sinfully yummy flavors. These can be your new favourite over the conventional hot wings! If you are not a fan of blue cheese, then no issue. Just substitute a few drops of fat free ranch dressing and there you go." Makes 24 Cups.

NUTRITION INFORMATION PER CUP:

70 calories | 4.6 g carbohydrates | 2.7 grams fat | 6.5 grams protein

INGREDIENTS

- 2-3 boneless, skinless chicken breasts

- 2 Tbsp. Olive oil

- 1/2 tsp. smoked paprika

- 1/2 tsp. chili powder

- 24 wonton wrappers

- 1 Tbsp. Butter, melted

- 1/2 cup Hot hot sauce

- 1/2 cup Blue cheese crumbles

- 3 scallions, sliced thinly

DIRECTIONS:

1. Preheat Oven to 350F degrees.

2. Brush Chicken breasts with olive oil, and then sprinkle evenly with smoked paprika and chili powder. Put in a skillet and cook for 20-30 minutes, or until the heart is no longer pink and the juices run clean. Remove chicken and let cool, then shred.

3. Meanwhile, Match a wonton wrapper into each of 24 miniature baking cups, then pressing on the wrappers closely but firmly to the sides of the cups. (Be careful to maintain the corners of each wonton wrapper available; differently, you won't be able to fill them) Bake for 5 minutes until very lightly browned. Maintain wontons in baking cups.

4. In a medium-sized bowl, stir together the melted butter and hot sauce. Add the chicken and stir fry until well coated. Then fill each wonton cup using a tbsp or two of chicken, then top with a pinch of cheese. Return wonton cups oven and cook for an additional 5-10 minutes, or till cheese is soft and melty. Remove and top with chopped scallions, and serve hot. These are best served immediately.

Boom Bang-a-Bang Chicken Cups

Coronation Chicken is a Royal dish lin Good Brittain Generally consisting of cooked poultry meat using an easy curried mayonnaise dressing table. For how easy the recipe is it is kind of amusing how it made its way on the feast menu to the coronation of Queen Elizabeth II in 1953. Nonetheless, it's delicious albeit easy...

These person lettus cups reveal the original character of Coronation Chicken however in healthful single portions. Enjoy!

NUTRITION INFORMATION PER CUP:

176 calories | 6 gram carbohydrates | 10 grams fat | 16 grams protein

INGREDIENTS

• 100g smooth peanut butter

• 140g Full-fat coconut milk or natural yogurt blended with 2 tablespoons desiccated coconut

• 2 tsp Sweet chili sauce

• 2 tsp soy Sauce

• 2-3 Spring onions finely painted

• 3 cooked skinless chicken breasts, shredded

• Two Baby Gem lettuces, large leaves split

• 1/2 Cucumber halved lengthways, seeds scraped out with a tsp, cut into matchsticks

• toasted Sesame seeds, for instance

DIRECTIONS:

1. On your smallest pan, lightly warm peanut butter, yogurt, 3

tablespoons water, candy chili, and soy sauce until melted together into a smooth sauce. Set aside and allow cooling.

2. Mix the Spring onions and chicken to the sauce and season. Chill before the celebration. Maintain the lettuce leaves and cucumber under moist kitchen paper.

3. To build, Add a package of lemon to each lettuce leaf cup, and a spoonful of the chicken mix. Sprinkle with sesame seeds sit on a huge platter for all to dig. Or just serve a heap of lettuce leaves alongside bowls of chicken and pineapple.

Ancho Chile Ground Beef Tacos

Street tacos Are Typically fried in oil and comprise fatty Variations of meat with veggies sauteed in oils. This causes some seriously high fat (little) tacos that make you hungry and needing additional food. That is no good once you're limiting calories to weight reduction. Satiety and decent nourishment is the title of this sport.

This edition of beef tacos will assess each the boxes. The Usage of lean ground beef and seasonings for taste keeps the calorie count low as well as the taste high.

NUTRITION INFORMATION PER TACO (4 ounce) :

171 calories | 5 grams carbohydrates | 6 grams fat | 25 grams protein

INGREDIENTS

- 1 tablespoon. ancho chile powder

- 1/2 tbsp. cumin

- 1/2 tsp. smoked paprika

- 1/2 tbsp. oregano

- 1/2 tbsp. garlic powder

- 1/2 tbsp. onion powder

- 1/2 tsp. coriander

- 1/2 tsp. salt

- 1/2 tsp. pepper

- 1 pounds. 95% Lean ground beef

- 1/3 cup water

- 1/2 tbsp. cornstarch

DIRECTIONS:

1. Mix Collectively ancho chili powder, cumin, paprika, oregano, garlic powder, onion powder, coriander, salt, and pepper. This produces a tasty homemade taco seasoning.

2. Brown that the Beef (or turkey) at a skillet until cooked through. Drain any excess fat. If you prefer you can add veggies in this step you can -- diced onions, yellow and red peppers, drained and canned diced tomatoes, or diced zucchini are yummy. Beans are also a tasty addition.

3. Whisk collectively the water and cornstarch. Increase the pan together with the taco seasoning and bring to a simmer. Let simmer for 3-4 minutes until sauce thickens.

Garlic Lemon Shrimp Kabobs

Kabobs are the greatest single-serving food. You understand How much you put on the skewer and every skewer is its serving. It will not get much easier than that. Using lean foliage creates this recipe standout since its essentially pure protein and calculable.

Add them into a salad or eat them on their own -- either way, these can keep you on course together with your regular diet!

NUTRITION PER KABOB (6 ounce) :

189 calories | 2 gram carbohydrates | 7 grams fat | 31 grams protein

INGREDIENTS:

• 1.33 pounds shrimp, peeled and deveined

• Salt and pepper

• 2 tablespoon Butter, melted

• 1/4 cup freshly squeezed lemon juice

• 4 tsp garlic, minced

• 1 teaspoon Italian seasoning

• 2 tablespoon Parsley, sliced

DIRECTIONS:

1. Preheat the oven to 450 degrees or preheat the grill.

2. Insert the Butter into a small saucepan. When it melts, add the garlic, lemon juiceand curry. Cook for 2-3 minutes until garlic is fragrant.

3. Twist the fish on skewers. Season with pepper and salt. To cook in the oven, then put on a baking sheet, and cook for 5-6 minutes until pink and cooked through. To cook on the grill, put right on the grill and cook for 2-3 minutes each side until opaque and cooked through.

4. When the Shrimp is cooked, brush together with the garlic butter mix and serve.

The Bottom Line:

While bariatric surgery isn't the "simple way" as a few people Think, you ought to be loving life! Enjoying life to the extreme entails enjoying calcium-rich food. The aim for life after bariatric surgery must be to boost your health, but also enjoying life.

Obviously, the life requires discipline and Dedication, therefore use these recipes to remain on your path to anew you" and steer clear of dull, tasteless food!

IMMEDIATE POST BARIATRIC SURGERY DIET: FLUIDS

There are 3 basic stages of ingestion after weight-loss Surgery, irrespective of type. 'FLUIDS', the very first, is frequently regarded as the most difficult. Many come home from surgery, feeling somewhat uncomfortable, certainly exhausted, clutching their clinic guidelines then hover from the kitchen uncertain about what to eat or drink following.

What to do? First of All, follow your physician and Bariatric group's advice to the letter. Some surgeons will urge clear then complete fluids for only a couple of days after surgeryothers for as long as 4 months. This will be to minimise digestion, so reduce the creation of waste and ensure maximum recovery of your gastrointestinal system.

'CLEAR LIQUIDS', the kind you can see that will comfortably travel up a straw, are on the schedule. They ought to be sipped slowly rather than gulped. It's necessary to get enough of these to stay hydrated, which actually means you will nearly always have one in your side from the first days. It's necessary that a number of these are 'supplements' to offer you a bit of nourishment.

Listed below are some typical great choices and you'll find Favorites one of them. What exactly does taste strange to start with, frequently too sweet, therefore dilute with ice or water to get a more acceptable flavour and concentration. It needs to be stated that number helps, ring the changes frequently so that boredom does not set in. Though there's a limited choice that is for a reason. They'll maximise recovery and you need to just move onto another phase when informed and prepared to achieve that.

General guidelines are that you must target for 2.5 to 3.5 Litres every day. It'll be quite tough to make this happen initially but do attempt. Spread them out equally. Everybody has distinct fluid requirements; the very best method to check you're well hydrated will be to have a look at the color of the urine. If output is light, you're drinking enough. When it's dark e.g. straw-coloured or darker or when there's minimal urine, then you want to drink more.

The recommended fluid portion size at any given time is usually believed to be less than 200 ml. At the very early days that this may look to be an enormous volume! Each beverage can be best taken more than one hour apart.

NEVER HAVE FIZZY DRINKS.

Fantastic CHOICES OF CLEAR FLUIDS

• Water

• Tea -- Warm conventional, herbal or fruit teas

• Java -- Warm, ideally light-hearted

• 'no-added-sugar' Or'sugar-free' squashes and cordials

• Bovril, Marmite or Oxo'salty' beverages diluted well with warm water

• sugar-free ice lollies

• sugar-free Jelly, composed according to packet directions

• Chicken, Beef or vegetable bouillon/broth/consommé or soup

• a whey Protein isolate fruit beverage such as Syntrax Nectar, composed with water --excellent for obtaining protein in the first days

Along with A DAILY MULTI-VITAMIN AND CALCIUM SUPPLEMENT

It may Look like an age but you'll reasonably quickly then Proceed on the'FULL LIQUIDS' phase which offers a bit more variety and nutrition to your dietplan. This is a very important stage because it prepares your own surgically-altered gut for longer food. This phase again may last only a couple of days or a couple of weeks based on surgical opinion. Always follow your surgeon's time-line.

Full liquids are the Ones that are believed smooth and pourable. Mix and match them with clear fluids to get great hydration during the day. Taste and flavour might still be off skew but variety is the secret to moving sensibly through this point and preparing your body for another one. It will get better each day and good customs could be immediately established at this point to reap dividends after.

Fantastic CHOICES OF FULL LIQUIDS

• milk Skimmed, semi-skimmed, soya, almond and Flora Guru active

• Milky Chai kind tea -- lightly-spiced for extra flavour

• Unsweetened Plain yogurt or yogurt with no additional sugar and fruit pieces

- Eloquent Cream-style (although not large fat) soups

- Whey Protein isolates beverages, hot, cold or freezing composed with milk or water

- Whey Protein isolates powder blended with milk or water and made in a ice cream

- Mashed Curry blended with a little soup or broth until lean and soup-like

- diluted Fruit juice

- Tomato or V8 juice -- warm or chilled

- Oatly -- Oat-based milk beverage

- Rice Fantasy first milk

- Slimfast Shakes and sauces, though Slimfast might prove too high in sugar for many skip patients

- Home-made Smoothies (although not too thick) and also shop-bought ones e.g. Innocent Strawberry and Banana, diluted if necessary using water

- Cocoa (created with 4 gram powder along with 200 ml semi-skimmed milk)

- Smooth-type cup-a-soups

- Highlight/Options Hot chocolate beverages

- Home-made Vegetable, poultry or fish broth, pureed until smooth and simmer into a smooth gliding consistency (slowly increase the depth as you advance through this point to the upcoming tender or pureed food phase)

- Low-fat and low-sugar custards

- Very gently put egg custards

MEDIUM TERM POST BARIATRIC SURGERY DIET: SOFT FOODS

If You Don't experience any Issues with the Phase 1 'Fluids' regime then you'll immediately move onto the next phase which comprises smooth, pureed, tender and crispy food, typically known as the'SOFT FOOD' phase.

This stage is generally followed for approximately 2-6 weeks after Surgery, though again consistently follow your bariatric group's information on when to begin and when to proceed.

Start gradually and make sure first your food choices Are loose and soft -- first phase baby food feel is what you're aiming for this. Progress to foods which may be easily crushed with a fork or blended to some'slurry' using milk, sauce or sauce. Do not be put off if something does not match...try it a couple of days later. Paradoxically a few days something goes down readily and the next time it does not. Learn how to listen to your own body and its own signs of gratification or angry.

You will still have to be aiming for at least 2 minutes of Liquids every day as well as those little 'foods'. Do not drink for 30 minutes before and 30 minutes afterwards and goal for 4-6 little 'meals' daily.

Eat slowly and the moments you're complete STOP EATING! Only one Extra tsp of food may send your own body into overload and there's not any nice way of stating this...what went down will return up or make you feel really uncomfortable! Recall that your new stomach pouch is simply about the size of an egg cup.

You may find it very suitable to suspend soft foods in ice Cube trays for this particular point. We discovered a stash of them, ready ahead of surgery, so beneficial in the forthcoming weeks. Foods in this type can be ready quickly for serving, variety is guaranteed as opposed to the constant round of this same-old and wastage is reduced to a minimal.

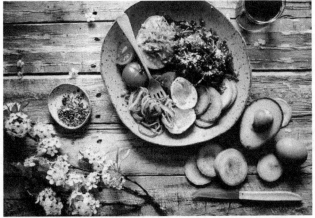

Listed below are some Fantastic food choices to your 'Soft Food' stage. Introduce these foods slowly replacing them since the days progress with ones which have more feel and flavour. Attempt to have 3 meals every day (ramekin or small tea plate dimensions).

Crispy foods, that will fall to pieces in water, for example Melba Toast, crispbreads, cream crackers and bread sticks may also be released from the latter times of Phase 2. Chew them completely before reduced to a smooth puree on your mouth. Do not confuse them for crispy foods e.g. salad and fruit that would cause difficulties at this point.

This is the point I think you Should Really Begin searching at preparing your recipes from scratch, so this way you understand just what's inside them. A lot of processed foods and prepared type foods have hidden fats and sugars to make them taste great but may be a banana skin to your weight loss surgery patient. Try out a few straightforward recipes to start with or be additional vigilant at ridding the trunk of pack nutrient advice of a food. You are aiming for low carb (as a rule than 3 percent fat i.e. less than 3 g per 100 gram recorded). In terms of sugar toleration levels fluctuate dramatically but I would not venture outside of the 6-7 gram struck per portion. It's believed that at levels past 10-15 gram you've got a strong probability of bypassing and sleeve 'dumping' syndrome and it will not assist those using a gastric group to maintain their calorie count reduced.

Fantastic CHOICES OF SOFT FOODS

• Weetabix, Porridge, Ready Brek having lots of skimmed or semi-skimmed

Milk to create a runny consistency

• mashed Banana with a small yogurt if enjoyed or using a low-carb and low-sugar custard

• Very soft cooked scrambled egg

• Finely Minced or grilled chicken or turkey in sauce

• pureed Fish at a thin sauce

• pureed canned fish e.g. tuna, pilchards, salmon or mackerel in a thin tomato

Sauce

- Soft and Smooth low-fat pate or distribute

- Plain Low-carb cottage cheese

- pureed Mashed potato and lean gravy

- pureed canned and extremely tender boiled vegetables like carrot and

Cauliflower

- Low-fat and low-sugar fromage frais

- Mild and Smooth low-carb and low-sugar mousse made with milk

- Heated Mashed potato mixed with grated low-fat cheese or low-fat lotion

Cheese

- milky Pudding like tapioca, sago or rice keep sugar into a minimum

- pureed Cauliflower cheese at a low-carb cheese sauce

- Pureed, Thickened or tender bit vegetable and poultry soups

- pureed casserole and stew dishes of a thinnish consistency

- Very Gently soft and cooked simple omelette

- poached Egg or even a soft-boiled one

- tender Beans, peas and lentils, pureed or simmer to get a small feel

- Thick fruit smoothies

- pureed Avocado

- Tiny Parts of home-cooked or ready-prepared and pureed main dishes

Like cottage pie, shepherd's pie, fish pie, fish-in-sauce, mild chilli con carne

Or their vegetarian choices created with quorn

- Low-sugar sorbets

- silken or smooth tofu

- crispy foods like crispbreads, Melba Toast, cream crackers and breadsticks

Long Term Post Bariatric Surgery Diet

Long-term POST BARIATRIC SURGERY DIET: THE FUTURE/FOOD FOR LIFE

Just when You're able to endure a Fantastic variety of foods From Phase 2, in the event you move tentatively onto Phase 3...ingestion FOOD FOR LIFE. Typically this happens between 8-16 weeks but everybody differs and constantly follow the recommendation of your very own bariatric team (and, simply since your dietician states you can eat grilled chicken, does not imply you can be able to do it straightaway, it sometimes requires a couple of times and retry events before you're ready to tolerate a specific food indefinitely). This is actually the point at which you ought to have the ability to attempt to consume an assortment of solid food, in tiny quantities. Consider with a side plate or kid's plate for a principle for serving size.

Foods to start with should possess a moist and soft feel so May need to be served with just a small sauce, cauliflower, sausage or dressing in order that they chew right into a moist mouthful, but as time goes onto a dryer texture is encouraged to get constriction and an perfect transition through the recently modified digestive system. These so-called 'slider' foods aid in the first days but may indicate that you're able to consume more in a subsequent stage only whenever you're searching to get 'satiety' and do not need foods to pass through the gut or pouch too fast. Gradually cut them down as you progress from week to week.

This is not a diet with a start and an end, nor is there Requirement to get a rush into the tape to reach a'goal weight', take it gradually, learn to recognise when you're filled and satisfied and do not eat beyond there of satisfaction. As time goes on gastric bypass and sleeve patients may learn to Recognise this stage and gastric group patients will surely, over time, find their 'sweet spot'.
It makes Great sense to cook Foods for everyone in the Household Instead of different ones for everybody at this stage. Why be a servant to a different regime which will thankfully suit all? Everybody can benefit from the foods appropriate here, higher protein, low fat and reduced sugar. Insert an excess accompaniment for all those growing members of their family members or a candy treat from time to time to acquire a perfect equilibrium.

THE REGIME AND SOME RULES

HIGH PROTEIN, LOW FAT AND LOW SUGAR IS THE MANTRA

• Consistently Consume your PROTEIN FIRST (the beef, eggs, poultry, fish) in your plate, then proceed onto the veggies and fruit and eventually the carbohydrate part -- potatoes, rice, rice.

• Pick LEAN PROTEIN with almost any visible fat removed (e.g. chicken skin); target for LOW FAT (you won't always manage it again aim for under 3 grams fat per 100g); and consistently opt to get a minimal SUGAR edition of a meal or foodstuff (the syndrome called 'dumping' -- see page 00, is believed to happen when you consume between 7 and 15 grams sugar in 1 hit).

• Eat 3 Meals daily with two or three little snacks if needed. These should meet you. However beware of creating a 'grazing' eating routine of little snacks every day.

• Eat Wholesome, strong food. Soft food definitely slips down more readily but you may wind up eating more over the duration of daily. If your food is drier and stronger you'll normally consume less complete and stay fuller for longer.

• EAT SLOWLY and cease once you feel complete. Take miniature bites and chew every piece 10-25 times. CHEW, CHEW, CHEW AND CHEW more! As soon as you're feeling complete STOP! Gone are the times when you have to clean your plate.

• Maintain your Fluid ingestion. It's also a fantastic idea to not drink immediately prior to, during or after a meal so that your stomach is not complete from fluids. Get into this habit once possible of not carrying food and fluids collectively.

• Take your Multi-vitamin, calcium as well as some other supplement regular religiously... they will make certain you have the very best chance of obtaining all of the extra nutrition you need that might not be provided in the low amount of food you're eating.

• The Hardest nutritional supplement to stay on course with is unquestionably protein. Aim for 70 grams every day. Quite tough to start with and do contemplate a protein isolate powder in the event that you regularly fall short. A spoonful of the powder in food or as a beverage can easily and economically provide 25 gram or a third of your needs at one fell swoop!

CAUTIONARY FOODS

There are some cautionary solid foods, Which Might not be Tolerated in the long and short term. Proceed with care when ingesting them:

• Non-toasted Bread, particularly white and soft

• Over-cooked pasta and boiled rice

• Red meat using a fibrous feel like beef and chops

• Stringy Vegetables such as green beans

• sweetcorn, Lettuce and pineapple with a toughened texture

• Pips, Skins and seeds from vegetables and fruit

• Dried fruits

• No Caution, only a straight no to carbonated beverages and chewing gum (for life)

Conclusion

Gastric sleeve is a sort of bariatric surgery, also referred to as weight loss surgery. It's sometimes suggested for men and women that are extremely overweight, or who have health problems brought on by obesity. You should only consider gastric sleeve surgery after attempting choices. The very first step is typically to test modifications to your food consumption as well as your everyday exercise and activity. Additionally, there are some medications which could help people eliminate weight. Surgery is usually considered just after these other choices are tried. Slimming down after gastric sleeve surgery can help reduce issues with type two diabetes, diabetes episodes and blood pressure, also will help improve heart health. After the surgery, you are going to begin with liquid foods. During the upcoming few weeks you may change to pureed food, then to food. Your meals will be a lot smaller and you might need to quit drinking with meals because of your little stomach. You'll have to make substantial lifestyle changes following bariatric surgery to eliminate weight and keep it off. By way of instance, you are going to receive nutritional advice from a dietitian about the best way best to modify your eating habits to stay healthy while losing weight. Your foods will be a lot more compact than previously. And you're going to likely take vitamins or supplements for life. You'll also need to, and also be in a position to, raise the amount of physical activity that you do.

CPSIA information can be obtained
at www.ICGtesting.com
Printed in the USA
BVHW011450110121
597543BV00001B/10